T0296919

Complementary Health Approaches for Occupational Therapists

Complementary Health Approaches for Occupational Therapists

Brittany Ferri, MS, OTR/L, CPRP

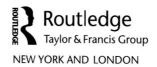

Routledge
Taylor & Francis Group
NEW YORK AND LONDON

Complementary Health Approaches for Occupational Therapists includes ancillary materials specifically available for faculty use. Included are an Instructor's Manual and PowerPoint slides. Please visit http://www.routledge.com/9781630918576 to obtain access.

Cover Artist: Christine Seabo

First published in 2021 by SLACK Incorporated

Published 2024 by Routledge
605 Third Avenue, New York, NY 10158

and by Routledge
4 Park Square, Milton Park, Abingdon, Oxon OX14 4RN

Routledge is an imprint of the Taylor & Francis Group, an informa business

© 2021 Taylor & Francis Group

Brittany Ferri *has no financial or proprietary interest in the materials presented herein.*

Library of Congress Cataloging-in-Publication Data

Names: Ferri, Brittany, author.
Title: Complementary health approaches for occupational therapists /
    Brittany Ferri.
Description: Thorofare, NJ : SLACK Incorporated, [2021] | Includes
    bibliographical references.
Identifiers: LCCN 2020027202 (print) | ISBN 9781630918576 (paperback)
Subjects: MESH: Occupational Therapy--methods | Complementary Therapies |
    Occupational Therapists
Classification: LCC RM735.3 (print) | NLM WB 555 |
    DDC 615.8/515--dc23
LC record available at https://lccn.loc.gov/2020027202

ISBN: 9781630918576 (pbk)
ISBN: 9781003523246 (ebk)

DOI: 10.4324/9781003523246

Additional resources can be found at
www.routledge.com/9781630918576

DEDICATION

To my rock, John, whose constant support not only made this project possible, but successful. To my most fervent fan and best friend, Rebecca, who was bragging about me long before I accomplished anything notable. To my mother, Linda, who encouraged my countless hours of reading and writing as a youth. To my father, Robert, who wanted to order *Hooked on Phonics* before I was even born, just to be safe. Thankfully, we can return the set in its original shrink wrap!

From the bottom of my heart, thank you all.

CONTENTS

Complementary Health Approaches for Occupational Therapists includes ancillary materials specifically available for faculty use. Included are an Instructor's Manual and PowerPoint slides. Please visit http://www.routledge.com/9781630918576 to obta in access.

ABOUT THE AUTHOR

Brittany Ferri, MS, OTR/L, CPRP is an occupational therapist and founder of Simplicity of Health, LLC, where she offers wellness consulting, health education for children and adults, health writing, and individual client treatments using holistic methods.

She has clinical experience in cognitive rehabilitation, psychiatric rehabilitation, complementary and alternative modalities, and teletherapy. Her nonclinical experiences have included roles such as medical writer, adjunct professor, and project coordinator. Ferri has also published *Effective Occupational Therapy Documentation*, a textbook for occupational therapy students and new therapists.

Ferri received her Master of Science in occupational therapy from Quinnipiac University in 2016. She is passionate about education, health promotion, and disease prevention for all of her clients and community partners. For more information, visit www.simplicityofhealth.com.

INTRODUCTION

My passion for health education has been lifelong since I have always been interested in learning the intricacies of health along with what makes our bodies tick. There are so many aspects of anatomy and physiology that we take for granted and expect to simply *work* each day.

This can be seen when someone catches the common cold. This may be unavoidable in certain circumstances, especially for someone who works in a hospital or in childcare. Yet, too often, something as trivial as congestion can be prevented by taking better care of our bodies. This annoyance may occur due to changes in sleep schedules, seasonal changes, an increase in stress, or deviation from a healthy diet.

A cold can be easy to prevent if we remain attentive to hand hygiene, receive our flu vaccinations, maintain a balanced diet along with regular exercise, and get the recommended amount of sleep each night. For most people, some of these aspects of a healthy lifestyle can fall by the wayside in lieu of a busier schedule or obligations that we prioritize.

The mention of small ways to prevent the common cold is not to guilt those individuals who are not maintaining healthy habits. Rather, this is intended to encourage the use of small lifestyle choices to prevent some large-scale health issues from arising. Stress is a large contributing factor in the development of many diseases and chronic conditions. The use of most complementary health approaches (CHA) can manage stress on a daily basis while often providing the body and mind with additional benefits.

If individuals become educated on the accurate use of these methods and their verified benefits, we can aim to change the landscape of health management. A more dedicated integration of CHA within health care can help to promote health as a part of daily life rather than primarily focusing on care for those who are already ill.

As vital as health education is for individuals within the community, it is even more integral for our fellow health care practitioners, including all types of therapists. In order to effectively promote health within the communities we serve, we must remain steadfast in our own understanding and education of these same concepts. In health and medicine, there is an incredible amount of debate between fact and fiction, myth and truth, and evidence-based research and mere claims, especially regarding CHA.

This book is intended to guide students and professionals alike in their journey toward continuously learning about stress, health, and daily management. These concepts can not only be applied to their patients and each individual they serve, but also their own lives. While education and awareness are paramount in the promotion of health, the applied and practical use of methods for improving health can also further the incorporation of CHA within each individual's personal health routine.

PART I

The History of Medicine

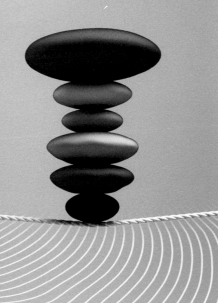

CHAPTER 1

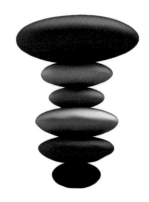

Definitions

The current state of medicine is largely different than it was just 20 short years ago. It is often said that one of the only constants in health care is change. This change has benefited some individuals more than others and can be likened to another constant in the world of health care: Individuals will always seek relief from what plagues them and will likely turn to some form of medical care for that relief.

Bouts of sickness over the course of the average person's lifetime have caused people to explore options they may never have otherwise. One option growing in popularity is alternative medicine. There are many terms associated with alternative medicine, with most terms closely related and often confused. This has caused misnomers and myths about how and when this form of medicine should be used. In order to have a proper understanding of alternative medicine, it is important to be informed regarding both traditional and nontraditional schools of medicine.

Ferri, B. *Complementary Health Approaches for Occupational Therapists* (pp. 3-12).
© 2021 Taylor & Francis Group.

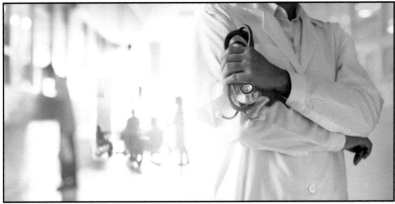

Figure 1-1. Allopathic medicine is the core of Western medicine. PopTika/Shutterstock.com

ALLOPATHIC MEDICINE

Allopathic medicine (Figure 1-1) describes the field of medicine that most people traditionally use and refer to when seeking medical care. This may also be referred to as *conventional* or *traditional medicine*. Allopathic medicine includes diagnostic methods, such as laboratory testing, heart monitoring, imaging (including X-ray, magnetic resonance imaging, computed tomography scan, ultrasound, and positron emission tomography scan), and strength tests. Treatment methods include prescription pharmaceuticals (including oral medication and intravenous infusion), surgery, radiation, lifestyle recommendations (sometimes), and referral to specialists or therapy practitioners, such as physical, occupational, and speech therapists. The most well-known practitioners of allopathic medicine are medical doctors, physician assistants, and doctors of osteopathic medicine. The main benefit of allopathic medicine is its use in treating immediate, life-threatening injuries and illnesses. It can be argued that pharmaceuticals are best at symptom treatment or suppression, rather than root-cause analysis and disease prevention. However, the general consensus is pharmaceuticals are another benefit of allopathic medicine (Shang et al., 2005).

ALTERNATIVE MEDICINE

Alternative medicine (Figure 1-2) is a term used to describe any medical treatment outside of allopathic medical treatment. Alternative medicine, also called *alternative modalities*, is a very broad term and can refer to thousands of treatment methods. Some of these methods are evidence-based and some are in the experimental stages. It is important to remember alternative medicine is used *instead* of allopathic medicine, hence it is an alternative option (National Center for Complementary and Integrative Health [NCCIH], 2018a).

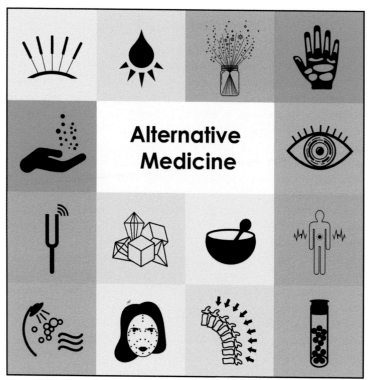

Figure 1-2. Alternative medicine includes a wide range of modalities. magic pictures/Shutterstock.com

Practitioners of alternative medicine vary largely based on the training and type of alternative medicine. For example, someone should possess a license and certification in acupuncture to ethically and legally practice acupuncture on patients. However, the title of someone practicing acupuncture may be oriental medicine practitioner, doctor of chiropractic medicine, or a range of other practitioners who have undergone the required training (National Certification Commission for Acupuncture and Oriental Medicine, n.d.). Due to the range of alternative medical treatments available, ascertaining the effects of alternative medicine as a whole is difficult. The benefits and purpose will vary based on the specific modality, model of care, and symptom(s) being addressed.

As with any health concept, it is important to stay well-informed regarding types of alternative medicine to determine the aspects that influence your practice as an occupational therapist. While alternative medicine refers to sole use of alternative methods for medical treatment, it is important to encourage patients to seek treatment from an allopathic medical doctor in instances of severe or life-threatening illness or injury.

COMPLEMENTARY MEDICINE

Complementary medicine describes medical practices used in conjunction with standard medical care. Complementary medicine, also referred to as *complementary modalities*, is similar to alternative medicine, as both are broad terms that can refer to nearly any method of care. Complementary modalities can be the same as alternative modalities, but the context where they are used is what sets them apart. The only difference between the two terms is whether or not conventional medical treatment is also being sought. Since complementary medical treatments are used *alongside* standard medical treatments, they may be self-implemented and self-monitored or monitored through a complementary medicine practitioner (NCCIH, 2018a). For example, a person may be managing anxiety by using anti-anxiolytic medication along with deep breathing exercises. In this instance, deep breathing techniques are considered a complementary modality.

The NCCIH says complementary modalities can be broken down into two categories: Natural products and mind and body practices (2018a). Natural products include vitamins, dietary supplements, and herbal blends or botanicals. Mind and body practices aim to join both the mind and body during an activity in order to achieve a calming effect. This includes, but is not limited to, yoga, meditation, tai chi, qigong, hypnotherapy, and relaxation techniques. The calming effect resulting from mind and body practices benefits those managing symptoms, such as anxiety, pain, stress, and depression. Improvements in the aforementioned symptoms can help relieve additional somatic complaints, such as sleep disturbances, appetite loss, weight gain, and inflammation (National Cancer Institute, 2018).

Most allopathic doctors treat patients who can benefit from complementary treatment. Similarly, most alternative medicine practitioners see patients who require treatment and monitoring from an allopathic doctor (Cohen, 2004). It is always recommended that patients seek treatment from an allopathic medical doctor in instances of severe or life-threatening illness or injury.

If patients have any questions about the use of complementary medicine alongside their allopathic treatment regimen, occupational therapists can provide education to the best of their ability. It is best practice to inform patients to seek further counsel from their doctor for questions that you were not trained or educated on.

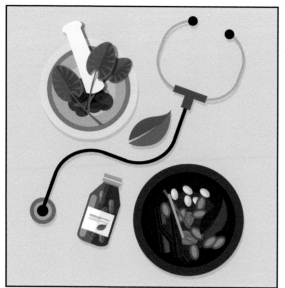

Figure 1-3. Integrative medicine takes a "whole-person" approach. Bakhtiar Zein/Shutterstock.com

INTEGRATIVE MEDICINE

Integrative medicine (Figure 1-3) describes a concept that treats the whole person by addressing the full range of physical, mental, emotional, spiritual, and environmental factors. Each of these factors has an impact on health, and all are treated through a collaborative relationship between patient and practitioner. Treatments based on an integrative medicine model are individualized to facilitate the innate response of the body to heal itself, with a large focus on health education and disease prevention (The Bravewell Collaborative, 2010). There are no specific treatments associated with integrative medicine, as it is simply a foundation any medical practitioner can use to guide the care of patients. Thus, integrative medicine can combine treatment methods in its attempt to address the whole person effectively. One of the main benefits of integrative medicine is its all-encompassing approach to medical care. This has assisted in removing the stigma associated with mental illness by addressing the mind and body in every session for every patient (Ross, 2009). An additional benefit of integrative medicine is the focus on the relationship of the patient and practitioner as a unit working toward individualized health. Integrative medicine also encourages the use of any treatment proven to be safe. This is also a major benefit that expands the possibilities for healing (Gade, 2018).

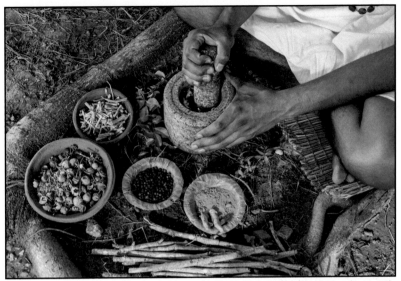

Figure 1-4. Ayurveda originated in India and has made its way to Western cultures. Nila Newsom/Shutterstock.com

As integrative medicine combines complementary medical care with allopathic medical care, treatments are implemented by a trained health care professional who can monitor a patient's response to all interventions. However, any treatments causing life-threatening symptoms should immediately be discontinued and brought to the attention of allopathic medical doctors.

Ayurvedic Medicine

Ayurvedic medicine (Figure 1-4) is one type of Eastern medicine originating from India. The diagnostic process of Ayurvedic medicine includes classification of a person's body and mind energies. There are three energies, or *doshas*, that may exist within a person. An Ayurvedic practitioner may identify an excess or deficiency in these doshas. Pitta, the dosha of fire, characterizes a person's metabolic abilities. Vata, the dosha of wind, is used to describe a person's mobility. Kapha, the dosha of water and earth, identifies the stability of a person's energies (Patwardhan et al., 2005).

Ayurvedic treatment includes diet and exercise recommendations along with health products. These health products can be plant-based, animal-based, metal-based, or mineral-based. Principles of Ayurveda include disease prevention through balance of the environment, body, and mind (NCCIH, 2019). Treatments include yoga, herbal medicine, deep breathing, acupuncture, massage, meditation, and sound therapy (Victoria State Government, 2018). There is minimal evidence regarding the effectiveness of many

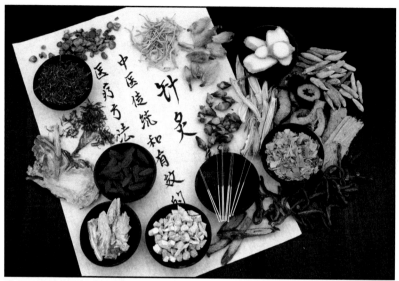

Figure 1-5. TCM focuses on balancing qi to avoid disease. marilyn barbone/ Shutterstock.com

Ayurvedic herbal remedies. However, Ayurvedic principles along with exercise- and meditation-based modalities are safe to use as complementary modalities if a patient is cleared for exercise by their doctor. It is always recommended that patients seek treatment from an allopathic doctor in instances of severe or life-threatening illness or injury.

TRADITIONAL CHINESE MEDICINE

Traditional Chinese Medicine (TCM) is another Eastern medicine that emphasizes each individual's connection to nature (Figure 1-5). TCM principles state that the absence of disease can be achieved through an adequate balance between all bodily energy forces, or *qi*. Two of these energy forces are yin and yang. Yin represents symptoms of cold and is characterized by ailments of the interior, including organs, bone marrow, internal energy, and blood. Yang represents symptoms of heat and is characterized by ailments of the exterior, including skin, hair, flesh, and energy meridians. Other energy forces include the five elements and are used to explain the stages of life and disease. These elements are fire, wood, metal, earth, and water. Disease can also result from an excess or deficiency in one of the seven emotions: Anger, fear, anxiety, fright, grief, pensiveness, and joy. Each of these emotions has a direct impact on the function of a corresponding organ that may cause disease (NCCIH, 2013b).

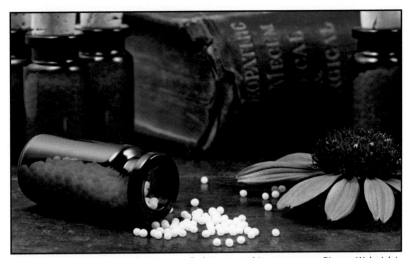

Figure 1-6. Homeopathy relies on small doses to achieve potency. Bjoern Wylezich/ Shutterstock.com

TCM diagnosis is based on inspection (looking), auscultation (listening), palpation (feeling), and inquiry (asking) in relation to each part of the body. Individualized treatments include herbal medicine, acupuncture, massage, cupping, and reflexology (Acupuncture and Massage College, 2017).

While benefits vary based on what treatments are provided, TCM is intended to alleviate symptoms of allergies, anxiety, joint pain, depression, rashes, and irregular menstrual cycles (NCCIH, 2013b). Despite its effectiveness in alleviating certain symptoms, there is still little evidence TCM can treat disease. It is always recommended that patients seek treatment from an allopathic doctor in instances of severe or life-threatening illness or injury.

HOMEOPATHIC MEDICINE

Homeopathic medicine (Figure 1-6), or *homeopathy*, is a German style of medicine based on two core principles. "Like cures like" refers to the idea that a disease-causing substance can provide relief when ingested in very small doses. Similarly, homeopathic medicine also states, "Less is more." This suggests the smaller the dosage taken, the more potent the substance will be in treating disease. Natural products used as homeopathic treatments are plant-based, mineral-based, and animal-based and intended for topical or oral use.

While there is limited evidence to support the sole use of homeopathy for the treatment of disease, the use of its principles can be combined with allopathic treatment (NCCIH, 2018b). Homeopathic medicine is intended to manage symptoms of allergies, migraines, depression, fatigue, joint pain, bowel dysfunction, and irregular menstrual cycles, along with minor abrasions and the common cold. There is minimal research on the effectiveness of homeopathy, as many believe the positive results from homeopathy are due to the placebo effect (Kiefer, 2016a). It is always recommended that patients seek treatment from an allopathic medical doctor in instances of severe or life-threatening illness or injury.

NATUROPATHIC MEDICINE

Naturopathic medicine, or *naturopathy*, is a European model of care that involves the use of the most natural treatment methods possible. The six principles of naturopathic medicine include firstly and always doing no harm, the use of nature as a healing power, the identification and treatment of the causes of disease, the treatment of the whole person, the prevention of disease, and the role of the doctor as a teacher (Association of Accredited Naturopathic Medical Colleges, 2017). Naturopathic diagnostic techniques are similar to that of allopathic medicine and may include laboratory testing, heart monitoring, imaging, and more. These diagnostic assessments are used to provide treatments, such as herbal and homeopathic products, manual or manipulative therapies, detoxification regimens, counseling, and diet- or exercise-based recommendations (NCCIH, 2017b).

The benefits of naturopathic medicine include relief from symptoms, such as allergies, headaches, infertility, indigestion, hormonal imbalances, joint pain, and fatigue. While naturopathic medicine is practiced by naturopathic doctors, patients may be directed toward allopathic doctors for severe or worsening symptoms (Kiefer, 2016b).

FUNCTIONAL MEDICINE

Functional medicine (Figure 1-7) is an approach rooted in biological identification of the core cause of disease. This approach is different than most other forms of medicine due to the idea that one condition can have multiple causes and one cause can result in multiple conditions. Functional medicine has foundations in nutritional science, genomics, and epigenetics. Diagnosis revolves around a detailed history of family, social, medical, and personal factors in order to link what are seemingly unrelated issues across an individual's life span. Functional medicine practitioners use the process of gathering, organizing, telling, ordering, initiating, and tracking symptoms to manage the care of each of their patients (The Institute for Functional Medicine, 2019). Interventions focus on modification of cellular systems to reverse the progression of disease in the gastrointestinal, endocrine, and immune systems. Functional medicine operates on the idea that almost all diseases stem from the structures and functions of these systems.

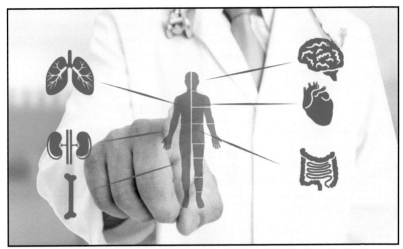

Figure 1-7. Functional medicine looks to the immune, gastrointestional, and endocrine systems to find the root cause of most diseases. Bjoern Wylezich/Shutterstock.com

Benefits of functional medicine include relief from symptoms, such as cardiovascular irregularities, hypertension, digestive issues, cognitive and neurological deficits, hormonal imbalances, skin abnormalities, elevated cholesterol, immune system deficiencies, and metabolic deficiencies (Cleveland Clinic, 2014). It is always recommended that patients seek treatment from an allopathic doctor in instances of severe or life-threatening illness or injury.

ENERGY FIELD MEDICINE

Energy field medicine, also known as *energy healing medicine*, involves the use of light touch to manipulate and rebalance the energies within the body. This is intended to restore imbalances that may be causing a range of physical or psychological ailments. One of the most common forms of energy field medicine is reiki. Like most other modalities in energy field medicine, reiki involves a practitioner directing their own energy through either light touch or by hovering their hands directly above the person. The collective intention of energy field medicine is to trigger a person's natural healing response by tapping into the body's innate abilities and energies.

There has not been much research on energy field medicine, reiki, or other energy healing modalities. However, reported benefits include a decrease in pain, inflammation, insomnia, depressive symptoms, and symptoms of anxiety (NCCIH, 2018c). As always, it is recommended that patients seek treatment from an allopathic medical doctor in instances of severe or life-threatening illness or injury.

Chapter 2

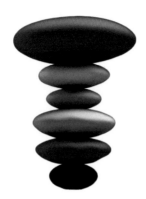

Complementary Health Approaches and Integrative Health in Practice

Complementary health approaches (CHA) and integrative health, previously known as *complementary and alternative modalities*, refers to any medical practice or product that is not part of conventional or allopathic, medicine (National Center for Complementary and Integrative Health, 2018a). The National Center for Complementary and Alternative Medicine identifies five classifications of CHA and integrative health: Alternative medical systems, mind-body techniques, biologically based treatments, manipulative and body-based practices, and energy therapies (2000). Mind-body techniques include any activity that focuses on the use of the mind to impact physical functioning. Manipulative and body-based practices involve the application of pressure to varying parts of the body to elicit a therapeutic response.

Occupational therapy (Figure 2-1) is defined by the American Occupational Therapy Association as "the therapeutic use of everyday life activities (occupations) with individuals or groups for the purpose of enhancing or enabling participation in roles, habits, and routines in home, school, workplace, community, and other settings . . . [these]

Ferri, B. *Complementary Health Approaches
for Occupational Therapists* (pp. 13-16).
© 2021 Taylor & Francis Group.

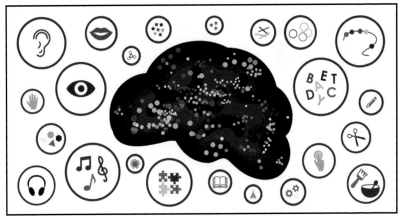

Figure 2-1. Occupational therapy interventions address deficits that are far beyond what meets the eye. magic pictures/Shutterstock.com

services are provided for habilitation, rehabilitation, and promotion of health and wellness for [patients] with disability- and nondisability-related needs" (2014). This definition points toward the individualized and holistic nature of occupational therapy as part of a health and wellness-based program. Occupational therapists can use any modalities, based in conventional medicine or CHA, in order to elicit occupational engagement. This is within an occupational therapist's scope of practice if the therapist is knowledgeable in the appropriate modality.

In light of an increase in CHA use, the American Occupational Therapy Association stated that these approaches "may be used within the scope of occupational therapy practice when they are used as preparatory methods or purposeful activities to facilitate the ability of [patients] to engage in their daily life occupations" (Giese, 2005). As with any treatment modality, occupational therapists must complete an evaluation and intervention plan to determine if the patient's deficits and needs warrant the use of CHA. To maintain ethical and client-centered care in accordance with the values of the profession, an occupational therapist must assess the patient's cultural traditions to determine if use of CHA is appropriate (Giese, 2005).

Some occupational therapy practitioners may use CHA in a manner that is technically outside of occupational therapy's scope of practice. This is acceptable only if the occupational therapist possesses the mandatory certifications and licenses to practice CHA with a primary concentration (Giese, 2005). For example, an occupational therapist with no additional certifications who incorporates CHA into their treatment must maintain focus on occupational engagement and functioning. On the contrary, an occupational therapist with additional certifications in a certain area of CHA may treat using any combination of modalities they choose, based on the patient's needs and the setting

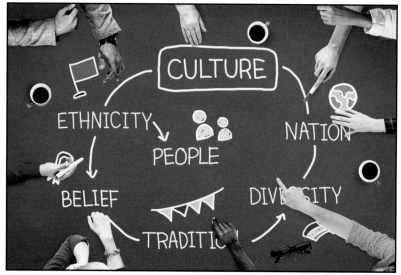

Figure 2-2. Cultural sensitivity should be the focus of all client-centered care. Rawpixel.com/ Shutterstock.com

where they are practicing. In a situation such as this, it is maximally important the occupational therapist consistently refers to their scope of practice, as well as state and third-party payer regulations to ensure compliance on all levels (Giese, 2005).

Due to recent evidence pointing toward cost reduction, market demand, and clinical effectiveness, some third-party payers now provide coverage for select CHA (Pelletier & Astin, 2002; Pelletier et al., 1999). This provides a growing foundation for the use of complementary approaches within the practice of occupational therapy.

Cultural competence (Figure 2-2) is an important factor that can either hinder or assist the implementation of CHA as part of occupational therapy treatment. A cultural context is defined as "customs, beliefs, activity patterns, behavioral standards, and expectations accepted by the society of which a [patient] is a member" (American Occupational Therapy Association, 2014).

These aspects of a cultural context, in some instances, may be strongly in favor of the use of CHA in the healing process. For example, a woman born in India who was raised in a traditional family may have been practicing yoga from a very young age, making her possibly more adept than an entry-level therapist. In this instance, bringing new adaptations to yoga can assist with strengthening and balancing the body. Similarly, education regarding safety awareness and contracting certain muscle groups while practicing yoga may be indicated. Her cultural context may serve to improve her treatment compliance, self-efficacy, and overall engagement in occupations.

In contrast, a patient's cultural context may impact a decision to forgo therapy altogether. For example, a child with oral-motor defensiveness and some problem behaviors may have been raised in a Jewish family with a rigid mealtime routine consisting of only certain foods and food combinations and no distractions while eating. Upon evaluation, an occupational therapist may want to sample different foods and begin each meal-time therapy session with meditation and visualization. The family may be resistant to this treatment and refuse to continue therapy due to their cultural beliefs. This family's cultural context has negatively impacted compliance, physical and emotional development, and independence as the child ages. In severe cases, cultural context may be a deciding factor in someone choosing to not receive even basic medical treatment of any kind. It is the duty of the occupational therapist to be mindful of and accommodating to the cultural needs of all patients.

These are just some examples of how CHA can be incorporated into occupational therapy practice. Additional scenarios include meditation for those with anxiety and depression; yoga for weakness, incoordination, or poor range of motion in any part of the body; deep breathing techniques for pulmonary disorders; and more.

CHAPTER 3

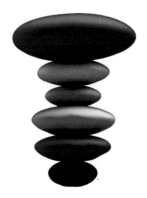

Working With Alternative Health Practitioners

An important part of effective multidisciplinary communication with alternative health practitioners in any setting is basic education on their scope of practice and benefits. Occupational therapists can add this information to their knowledge base in order to train and educate others on new disciplines. A supportive work environment and collaboration are both vital to smoothly integrate alternative health practitioners within an existing health care team. Mutual respect among roles is key, in addition to verifying quality outcomes of care (Nancarrow et al., 2013). It may be difficult to work with someone if you do not understand what their role is or if there are minimal positive results from their work.

Interdisciplinary and multidisciplinary work are large parts of a successful health care system. Most therapists have worked with, and are likely aware of the roles of, social workers, registered nurses, physical therapists, speech therapists, and medical doctors. While alternative health practitioners may hold some of these traditional titles, they likely hold additional certifications, too. The requirement for complementary health approaches certifications and licensures is largely dependent on

Ferri, B. *Complementary Health Approaches
for Occupational Therapists* (pp. 17-18).
© 2021 Taylor & Francis Group.

the modality practiced. Still, it is critical to know which credentials practitioners are warranted to hold, and what credentials are likely to be held by legitimate alternative health practitioners.

Licensure requirements will vary from state to state, and some professions may not require licensure at all. Many regulatory boards that govern certain modalities offer certifications to ensure adequate training. Knowledge of the specific requirements of each modality is crucial to gain an understanding of how alternative health practitioners function. Chapters addressing individual modalities will discuss credentialing further.

PART II

Complementary Health Approaches and Integrative Health

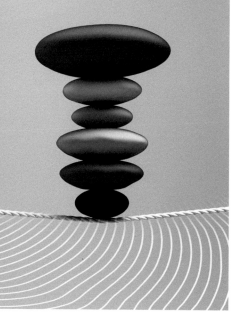

CHAPTER 4

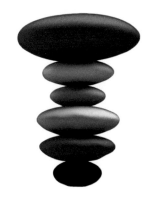

Disclaimers

As mentioned earlier, all complementary health approaches (CHA) can be used as alternative or complementary methods depending on their use, or lack thereof, with allopathic medicine. However, most all CHA are intended for use as complementary modalities as they do not address acute or life-threatening medical issues. Some of these may not be available for use by occupational therapists without additional certification. However, patients seen by allopathic doctors may be simultaneously seeing alternative health practitioners within the community. Therefore, it is important to understand what each modality is, how it is used, and any risks involved, especially any that may interfere with occupational therapy treatment.

As always, it is important to document all of this information to ensure the occupational therapist is keeping safety first and intending to do no harm. Occupational therapists should also document the counsel and education provided to patients regarding all modalities and conditions. This is both ethically and legally appropriate to minimize liability on the behalf of the occupational therapist.

Ferri, B. *Complementary Health Approaches for Occupational Therapists* (pp. 21-22). © 2021 Taylor & Francis Group.

There are no general CHA contraindications to keep in mind, as each modality may possess some contraindications while other modalities hold no restrictions. According to the laws of ethical practice, it is important to complete a thorough assessment of each patient before using any modality to prevent risk of injury. It is also your responsibility as a therapist to educate the patient on any potential hazards or risks.

Some modalities, often those offering certification and licensure, have specific guidelines on scope of practice. This becomes especially important when documenting and speaking about such modalities. For example, certain CHA state that practitioners do not attempt to assess, claim, counsel, cure, diagnose, evaluate, heal, mitigate, prescribe, prevent, make prognoses, recommend, repair, or treat. You may recognize some of these terms (such as prevent, counsel, treat, assess, and recommend) as being commonly used within occupational therapy practice, while diagnosis is strictly excluded from job functions as outlined in the scope of practice. Similarly, avoid all of the aforementioned terms when educating patients about CHA or while performing CHA on patients. This removes liability from the therapist regarding claims of healing, curing, or treating their symptoms or conditions. For more information about appropriate verbiage, it is important to thoroughly research a modality before using it in practice.

Each of the following chapters will detail contraindications, precautions, and potential side effects associated with each modality. When contraindications are present for a modality, the modality should not be performed on patients who meet those criteria. When precautions are present for a modality, performing the modality on a certain patient may increase their risk of an adverse side effect. When side effects are present for a modality, the modality may have the indicated reactions to any patient.

CHAPTER 5

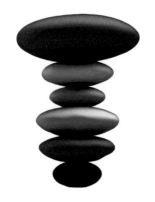

Acupressure

Traditional Chinese Medicine (TCM) has used acupressure as a modality for thousands of years. Acupressure uses fingers and thumbs to apply medium to firm pressure to specific points in the body (Smith et al., 2017). These points are to stimulate the flow of energy, or *qi*, in the body through channels called meridians (Figure 5-1). Applying pressure to these meridians aims to clear blockages in qi and increase circulation while stimulating the body's self-healing abilities (University of California at Los Angeles Integrative Medicine, 2019). Patients should be aware that acupressure is not a quick fix. Due to the need for sustained pressure on only one point at a time, it can take multiple, prolonged sessions to see results (Wong, 2017).

Acupressure is not used as a method of diagnosis; it is a technique associated with the practice of TCM. A practitioner of TCM may evaluate and determine the need for acupressure.

Ferri, B. *Complementary Health Approaches for Occupational Therapists* (pp. 23-27).
© 2021 Taylor & Francis Group.

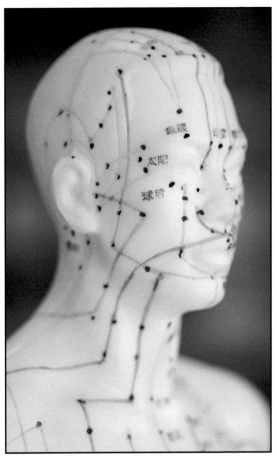

BENEFITS

Anecdotal evidence suggests acupressure can relieve muscle tension and pain, making it sought after by those who experience fatigue, migraines, menstrual cramps, motion sickness, and frequent nausea (Macznik et al., 2017; University of California at Los Angeles Integrative Health, 2019). Although acupressure may be practiced in an attempt to relieve anxiety and manage stress, there is little research supporting the use of acupressure for either mental or physical symptoms.

Contraindications, Precautions, and Side Effects

Acupressure is contraindicated in patients with osteoporosis or fractured bones in the healing stages. Acupressure should not be performed on pregnant women. It is also unsafe to use acupressure on patients with cancer, bleeding disorders, high blood pressure, or those taking anticoagulant medications. The pressure created by this modality can cause clotting or complications for patients with any of the above conditions. There are no known precautions or side effects associated with acupressure.

Credentialing

It is safe to perform simple acupressure after reviewing the associated risks and determining if they are applicable to your patients. If you are interested in providing acupressure to patients on a consistent and regular basis, certification is encouraged. The National Certification Commission for Acupuncture and Oriental Medicine states those who are interested can obtain certification as an Asian bodywork therapist by completing an approved training program and subsequently passing a certification exam (2018). For those with a license in massage therapy, many massage therapy schools also provide specialty training or elective courses in acupressure (National Certification Commission for Acupuncture and Oriental Medicine, 2018).

Acupressure and Occupational Therapy

Basic acupressure can be incorporated as a preparatory activity for patients who are free of any contraindications. Most mental health settings have the structure and freedom to integrate the basics of acupressure into occupational therapy treatments. Acupressure basics can be integrated into group therapy as a self-care tool or taught individually to patients needing more concentrated training.

Patients with cognitive deficits who are unable to learn the basics of acupressure may be given acupressure mats to use with supervision. Since acupressure mats do not isolate specific points on meridians, their benefits are not the same as those of standard acupressure. However, their size allows for consistent pressure to be provided over a larger portion of the body (e.g., buttocks and upper leg muscles or lower and mid-back muscles). For this reason, it can assist in temporarily relieving tense muscles.

BASICS OF ACUPRESSURE

Gallbladder 20: This point is located where the neck muscles insert at the lower skull. It is recommended to cradle the head using both hands and use both thumbs to massage the point. Acupressure at this point is recommended for relief of headaches, blurry vision, fatigue, and cold-like symptoms.

Gallbladder 21: This point is located at the clavicle bone, just above the anterior shoulder. Massaging these points by pinching the shoulder muscles is recommended to provide relief from stress, facial pain, headaches, tooth pain, and neck pain.

Large Intestine 4: This point can be found in the web between the thumb and second digit. Massaging this point for several seconds can assist with relief of stress, headaches, tooth pain, facial pain, and neck pain.

Liver 3: This point is located where the first and second metatarsal bones meet. Acupressure at this point is recommended for relief of stress, lower back pain, high blood pressure, limb pain, insomnia, and anxiety.

Pericardium 6: This point is located on the anterior forearm, several inches below the wrist. Palpation will find a point between tendons, which should be massaged. Acupressure at this point is recommended for relief of nausea, anxiety, carpal tunnel syndrome, motion sickness, headaches, and heart palpitations.

Triple Energizer 3: This point can be found at the base of the fourth and fifth metacarpals. Massaging this point is recommended for relief of temporal headaches, shoulder pain, neck tension, and upper back pain.

Spleen 6: This point can be found on the lower leg, several inches above the ankle in a depression under the tibia. Massaging this point is recommended for relief of urological and pelvic disorders, insomnia, and fatigue.

Stomach 36: This point is located on the lower leg, just lateral to the patella. Massaging this point is recommended for relief of fatigue, depression, knee pain, and gastrointestinal distress (University of California at Los Angeles Integrative Medicine, 2019).

CONSIDERATIONS FOR PRACTICE

This modality does not require the use of any equipment. Therapists should ideally implement acupressure in a quiet space, but there is no need for individuals to be in a large, spacious area. Individuals would most benefit from a semiprivate location to allow for focus and concentration. Acupressure does not require individuals to remove any articles of clothing, other than perhaps adjusting their sleeves or shirt necks to better access areas, such as the wrist, forearm, and clavicle. Individuals would benefit from visual models, either from therapist demonstration or through printed/virtual images. Therapists who have prior knowledge of a patient's main areas of concern can prepare specific sequences or routines that would benefit patients. However, therapists who have more experience in acupressure can devise patient routines on the spot based on issues that a patient reports or is currently demonstrating.

Therapists may write acupressure-related goals in some of the following areas:

- Becoming independent in the use of acupressure as a stress management tool
- Increasing education regarding the mind-body connection
- Remembering the sequence for a certain number of acupressure points
- Fine-tuning their force modulation to elicit the optimal response from each acupressure point
- Incorporating acupressure into a daily self-care routine

CHAPTER 6

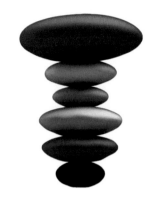

Acupuncture

Acupuncture is a modality that has been used as part of Traditional Chinese Medicine (TCM). Acupuncture involves the use of thin needles to puncture the skin at certain points on the body (Figure 6-1). These points are specific to the flow of energy, or *qi*, in the body through channels called meridians. Stimulating these points on the skin aims to clear blockages in qi and increase circulation while stimulating the body's natural healing response (University of California at Los Angeles Integrative Medicine, 2019). The use of herbs may also be added to this practice through moxibustion, which involves burning herbs above the skin to produce a thermal effect over certain acupuncture points (Figure 6-2).

Acupuncture is not used as a method of diagnosis; it is a technique associated with the practice of TCM. A practitioner of TCM may evaluate and determine the need for acupuncture.

Ferri, B. *Complementary Health Approaches for Occupational Therapists* (pp. 29-32). © 2021 Taylor & Francis Group.

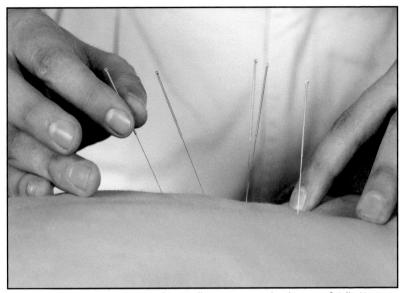

Figure 6-1. Acupuncture uses very thin needles to puncture the skin superficially. Nanette Dreyer/Shutterstock.com

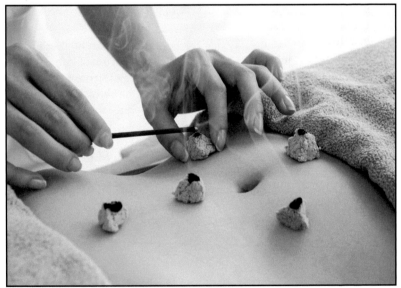

Figure 6-2. Moxibustion uses heat to burn herbs over certain meridian points. Leonardo da/Shutterstock.com

BENEFITS

Anecdotal evidence suggests acupuncture can improve lower back pain, addiction, and insomnia. Research shows acupuncture is effective in reducing joint pain, such as low back pain, neck pain, knee pain, and headaches (Berman et al., 2010; Chou et al., 2007; Hinman et al., 2014; Linde et al., 2009; Witt et al., 2006).

While acupuncture originally gained traction with the claim of assisting with smoking cessation, there is no evidence supporting its use for that purpose. There is also little evidence acupuncture benefits individuals with anxiety or depressive disorders, though this remains a technique to address emotional disorders in eastern countries.

CONTRAINDICATIONS, PRECAUTIONS, AND SIDE EFFECTS

When completed properly, there are no side effects resulting from acupuncture. Precautions are present for any patient who receives acupuncture following unsafe procedures, such as using nonsterile needles or improper technique. Adverse side effects associated with incorrect procedures include collapsed lungs, infection, punctured organs or blood vessels, and injury to the nervous system (National Center for Complementary and Integrative Health, 2016a).

Acupuncture is contraindicated in patients with impaired blood clotting, weakened immune systems, pacemakers, and abnormal or artificial heart valves. These patients should not receive acupuncture due to the risk of infection or puncture (De Groot, 2001).

CREDENTIALING

It is safe to perform acupuncture after reviewing the associated risks and determining if they are applicable to your patients. A state license is required to practice any acupuncture. Specific requirements will vary from state to state; however, all state acupuncture licenses warrant satisfactory completion of educational and examination requirements. The Accreditation Commission for Acupuncture and Oriental Medicine sets forth these standards and requires a minimum of 4,050 hours of classroom instruction and supervised clinical experience. The National Certification Commission for Acupuncture and Oriental Medicine administers examinations (2019).

ACUPUNCTURE AND OCCUPATIONAL THERAPY

For those occupational therapy practitioners who have a valid license to practice acupuncture, the ideal place to use this modality would be individual sessions within a private practice. Hospitals, nursing homes, and other traditional therapy settings have restrictions relative to safety, location, complexity of patient medical conditions, and methods of service delivery. This makes acupuncture a difficult modality to implement without the liberties of a private practice clinic space.

Occupational therapists who are dually licensed can combine acupuncture with other modalities, including lifestyle redesign, nutritional recommendations, health and wellness consulting, and many other complementary and alternative modalities.

CONSIDERATIONS FOR PRACTICE

Acupuncture requires therapists to have an ample supply of single-use, sterile needles for each patient session. Therapists should arrange for a private area where patients can comfortably remove articles of clothing as needed according to the body part where they will receive the acupuncture. Patients who are unfamiliar with or nervous about acupuncture should have additional amenities, such as soothing music, calming aromas, and comfortable blankets to promote a feeling of ease. Patients should receive written or verbal education on the risks of this modality and the benefits that they should experience. Therapists must provide individuals with continual instruction to ensure that patients maintain appropriate body positions and muscle relaxation throughout the process. Most therapists will develop a specific plan regarding what body part to perform the acupuncture on, but they can alter the plan if patients report increased pain, stiffness, or other symptomology.

Therapists may write acupuncture-related goals in some of the following areas:

- Adhering to planned and scheduled acupuncture sessions to improve health management skills
- Lowering pain levels
- Tracking symptoms before and after acupuncture sessions
- Understanding the risks and intended benefits of acupuncture

CHAPTER 7

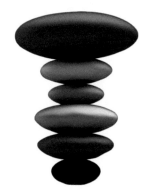

Animal-Assisted Therapy

The mere presence of animals can assist in providing enjoyment and relaxation to those with illness or recent injuries. Animal-assisted therapy (AAT) is the use of animals to assist in rehabilitating patients with acute or chronic injuries (Figure 7-1). AAT is not to be confused with pet therapy, which involves simply being around pets—typically dogs—in an effort to decrease loneliness and isolation. The use of animals can help patients achieve physical, mental, social, and emotional goals. Canines and equines are the animals most commonly used for therapy, though AAT can involve a variety of animals.

AAT is not a method of diagnosis, meaning therapists providing AAT must complete evaluations in their respective disciplines to determine a patient's weaknesses and areas of need. Then, AAT can address goals in these functional areas (American Addiction Centers, 2018).

Ferri, B. *Complementary Health Approaches for Occupational Therapists* (pp. 33-36). © 2021 Taylor & Francis Group.

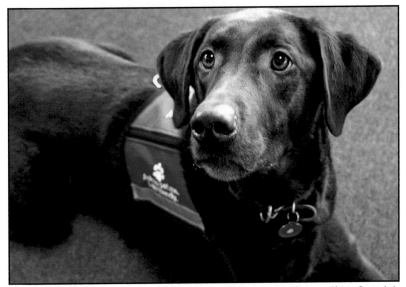

Figure 7-1. Dogs are some of the most popular animals to use in therapy. Shine Caramia/Shutterstock.com

Benefits

Some benefits of AAT are subjective, varying based on each individual's perception of and preference toward animals. Research has shown that AAT is effective in improving quality of life in older individuals with dementia, along with decreasing suffering of children receiving palliative care (Gilmer et al., 2016; Wood et al., 2017). AAT can also assist with decreasing symptoms of post-traumatic stress disorder and trauma survivors (Mims & Waddell, 2016).

While many benefits of AAT are psychosocial in nature, there is some research supporting the use of AAT in those with physical disabilities. Research has shown hippotherapy, or equine-assisted therapy, can help improve the symmetry of trunk movements in children with cerebral palsy (Mutoh et al., 2019).

Contraindications, Precautions, and Side Effects

Precautions associated with AAT include injury resulting from interaction with the animal, such as scratches, bites, or a fall related to tripping over the animal. Additional precautions are regarding poor sanitation and hygiene resulting from allowing animals into a hospital or skilled nursing facility. Having

AAT take place in a room not used for patient care or traveling to an outdoor portion on the hospital grounds can avoid the latter of these precautions.

AAT is contraindicated for patients with infectious diseases who are under strict contact precautions. AAT is also contraindicated for patients with a history of trauma related to animals, such as an attack or injury. AAT should not be used with patients who have allergies to the animal being used. While not a contraindication, it is important to be mindful that a side effect of AAT may be the patient developing an attachment to the animal resulting in difficulty terminating the therapeutic relationship.

CREDENTIALING

Pet therapy certification can be obtained if your current animal undergoes obedience and other training with the American Kennel Club. This will allow your pet to provide therapy in a variety of settings. It also provides basic training to the owners in relation to commands and safety in case of an emergency (American Kennel Club, 2015).

A license is not needed to practice AAT; however, a certification is required. Certification can be completed from several places, including the Animal Behavior Institute and the Animal Assisted Therapy Program of Colorado. There are no prerequisites to enter these programs, which include several training courses in addition to 40 hours of practical experience in the community (Animal Behavior Institute, 2017).

ANIMAL-ASSISTED THERAPY AND OCCUPATIONAL THERAPY

Therapists who complete the AAT certification can start their private practice, begin consulting, or add AAT interventions to services offered at their current place of work. AAT can take place in hospitals, skilled nursing facilities, school settings, outpatient clinics, and anywhere occupational therapy is provided.

AAT can be utilized as an individual- or group-treatment method for those patients who benefit from this modality. Mental health settings would benefit from leisure groups involving animals. However, the range of AAT is much larger than leisure. The psychosocial benefits can be incorporated into educational groups focused on self-esteem and emotional intelligence, skill-based trainings on social interaction and appropriate attachment, and functional trainings related to home management and caretaking.

CONSIDERATIONS FOR PRACTICE

Therapists using AAT should first identify whether a patient is well-suited to have animals incorporated into therapy. This can be determined by assessing factors such as preference, symptoms, behaviors, and overall disposition for therapy. Patients should work with specially trained animals under close supervision from a therapist while in an open space, preferably outdoors. Therapy can proceed only after patients understand basic etiquette for interacting with animals. Therapists should continually evaluate whether or not current patient weaknesses and goal areas are a good fit for intervention with animals. Therapists who use AAT in practice should be able to effectively control animals, ensure patient participation and safety, and offer adequate instruction for all parties involved. This may warrant the assistance of therapy aides or rehabilitation techs who have experience with animals.

Therapists may write AAT-related goals in some of the following areas:

- Improving range of motion, strength, endurance, coordination, and activity tolerance based on participating in therapeutic activities with animals
- Appropriately managing behaviors
- Increasing subjective quality of life
- Enhancing executive functions, such as sequencing, judgment, and memory
- Using appropriate social etiquette around animals
- Exercising good safety awareness
- Following predetermined rules
- Taking turns during activities with animals
- Using interactions with animals to manage uncomfortable emotions
- Self-advocating to adopt an emotional support animal or service animal

CHAPTER 8

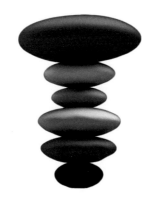

Aquatic Therapy

Aquatic therapy is a term used to describe a range of treatments provided in a water-based setting to assist in restoring, extending, and maintaining quality of function in individuals with acute or chronic illnesses. Water-based treatments include hydrotherapy, aquatic exercises, and spa therapy. Aquatic therapy may often be confused with aquatic fitness classes that have a focus on generalized wellness. Aquatic therapy can also be mistaken for adapted aquatics, or modified activities in a water-based environment for those with severe disabilities (Aquatic Therapy and Rehab Institute, n.d.).

Aquatic therapy can be used to improve range of motion for individuals with acute orthopedic diagnoses, those who have recently had surgery, and athletes requiring sports rehabilitation (Cleveland Clinic, n.d.). On the other end of the spectrum, aquatic therapy also can be used for individuals who have difficulty with standard exercises or activities on land. The properties of water allow for a lighter, more comfortable, and more tolerable pressure on the joints of the body. Water-based therapy gives a wider range of exercise options to those wishing to build strength

Ferri, B. *Complementary Health Approaches for Occupational Therapists* (pp. 37-41). © 2021 Taylor & Francis Group.

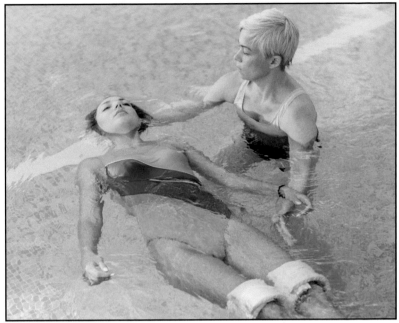

Figure 8-1. Trained therapists guide patients throughout entire aquatic therapy sessions. Liukov/Shutterstock.com

and endurance as part of rehabilitation (Cleveland Clinic, n.d.). Aquatic therapy can be practiced with individuals who do not know how to swim, as a trained instructor guides the entire session (Figure 8-1).

Benefits

An individual's ability to be buoyant in the water allows for relief of pressure on joints, increased oxygen flow to all parts of the body, and decreased stress on tissues and muscles, along with possible elimination of a patient's fear of falling. Water's buoyancy also allows therapists to easily handle weak or large patients (Aquatic Exercise Association, 2010).

Aquatic therapy has been demonstrated to improve balance and coordination, while decreasing pain in women diagnosed with fibromyalgia (Rivas Neira et al., 2017). Research has shown an improved quality of life in patients with multiple sclerosis who participated in regular aquatic therapy (Corvillo et al., 2017). Aquatic therapy has also slightly improved gait variability of patients with Parkinson's disease (Carroll et al., 2017).

Contraindications, Precautions, and Side Effects

Precautions related to aquatic therapy include risk of infection for improperly dressed wounds and drowning if an instructor leaves someone unattended. There are no known side effects associated with aquatic therapy.

Aquatic therapy is contraindicated for patients who experience seizures, have an allergy to chlorine, or have open pressure ulcers or other wounds. Aquatic therapy should also not be practiced on patients who are incontinent or have a fear of the water. Contraindications relative to specific aquatic therapy methods can be found in the section where techniques are discussed.

Credentialing

Aquatic therapists typically have licenses in physical therapy, occupational therapy, sports medicine, or athletic training. A license to practice rehabilitation is required in order to obtain certification as an aquatic therapy and rehabilitation instructor. Interested therapists should have 15 hours of education (not work experience) in aquatic therapy prior to entering the certification program. The certification program consists of three educational courses along with an exam (Aquatic Therapy and Rehab Institute, n.d.).

Aquatic Therapy and Occupational Therapy

Therapeutic professionals can practice aquatic therapy in most any setting with access to a large pool, or a pool with features making it ideal for use. Settings may include hospitals, outpatient centers, and sports fitness clinics. Aquatic therapy is mainly for the purposes of regaining movement, strength, and endurance, making it an ideal therapeutic exercise intervention. Therapeutic activities should complement aquatic therapy, along with simulated or real-time training of functional tasks for a complete intervention plan. See the next section for specifics and more contraindications for aquatic therapy techniques.

BASICS OF AQUATIC THERAPY

The Bad Ragaz Ring Method (BRRM) is a technique where the therapist assists the patient in maintaining a supported horizontal position (either supine or prone). Flotation devices are at the neck, pelvis, and knees or ankles. The therapist can position themself at any of the flotation devices to gently sway, rock, or roll the patient. By providing resistance, spinal elongation, and passive range of motion, the therapist is using neuromuscular re-education to assist in reducing tone.

BRRM assists with preparing patients for weight-bearing activities while decreasing tone and providing proprioceptive input. Contraindications specific to BRRM include frequent ear infections, due to the patient's immersion in the water.

Watsu, or watzu, is a technique that does not use any flotation devices and simply focuses on the therapist cradling the patient in the supine position. While rhythmically moving through the water, the patient is encouraged to coordinate their breath while various body parts are stretched. The therapist switches positions and cradles the patient in the reverse position to provide the same method to the opposite side. Watsu can be helpful for those patients who experience muscle guarding, low energy, cognitive and emotional deficits, muscle pain, and poor breathing patterns. Watsu is contraindicated in patients with range of motion restrictions in place as well as those who suffer from frequent ear infections and vestibular diagnoses.

Ai chi is another technique that assists with connecting the mind and body by emphasizing a focus on breathing, movement patterns, and posture while engaging in guided imagery and visualization. Patients completing ai chi stand in water at shoulder level while keeping a wide stance with toes out and knees slightly bent. Movements, such as uplifting, enclosing, folding, soothing, gathering, and freeing, include focus on the core muscles. Weight-shifting movements are slow and broad, using both the arms and legs. Being similar to tai chi, ai chi increases blood circulation, metabolism, body awareness, and balance. Ai chi is contraindicated in patients who continue to experience significant pain with movement.

AquaStretch is the last technique that focuses largely on effective pain management due to its ability to release scar tissue and other fascial adhesions. While in the corner of the pool, patients wear weights and make bodily adjustments in response to typical joint pressure. The buoyancy of the water allows patients to stretch for longer and higher ranges than they could tolerate on land.

(continued)

> ### BASICS OF AQUATIC THERAPY (CONTINUED)
>
> The basic steps of AquaStretch include playing, which allows for experimentation with painful positions, followed by freezing in that exact position and then allowing the therapist to apply pressure to the painful area. While the therapist is still applying pressure, patients are encouraged to make bodily adjustments if they would like. This results in small-scale movements that relieve pain. AquaStretch relieves muscle soreness and improves flexibility. Contraindications specific to AquaStretch are soft tissue injuries, fractures, and cognitive deficits that impact a patient from knowing the difference between "good pain" and "bad pain" (Aquatic Exercise Association, 2010; Brody & Geigle, 2009; Sova, 2012).

CONSIDERATIONS FOR PRACTICE

Occupational therapists who plan to use aquatic therapy should prepare their patients through therapeutic exercises and activities. While aquatic therapy is especially beneficial for patients who cannot tolerate movement against gravity, therapists must ensure that patients are making adequate progress in standard treatment methods and show sufficient motivation for aquatic therapy. Therapists should evaluate the environment where the therapy pool is located to guarantee its safety for all users. The individual assessment process should also consider patient sensitivities to noises, smells, and other stimuli as well as the ability to follow simple directions for maximum benefit from aquatic therapy. This means therapists may need to schedule appointments around cleaning schedules and peak pool times, while ensuring the availability of a second person to assist with transfers, if needed.

Therapists may write aquatic therapy–related goals in some of the following areas:

- Improving range of motion
- Increasing endurance
- Enhancing strength and activity tolerance
- Reducing edema
- Following directions
- Decreasing pain levels
- Increasing independence in transfers and functional mobility
- Utilizing safety awareness and judgment
- Managing difficult behaviors

CHAPTER 9

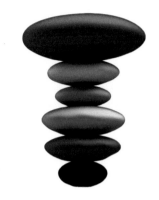

Aromatherapy

Growing in popularity among the general population, aromatherapy is one of the most common complementary modalities currently in use. Aromatherapy involves the use of essential oils from trees, herbs, or flowers (Figure 9-1). This modality is often combined with other complementary health approaches, such as therapeutic massage and acupuncture, to alleviate common symptoms.

Essential oils can be used in some of the following ways:

- Passive inhalation through a diffuser, nebulizer, or spray
- Direct inhalation from the bottle or a cup of hot water with the oil
- Mixed with a carrier oil for use in bath water
- Direct application or massage into the skin
- With some oils, ingestion in a cup of hot water for internal use

Due to differences in chemical makeup, there are specific usage instructions for each essential oil regarding absorption rates along with emotional and physical effects on the body. There are no U.S. Food and Drug Administration requirements on essential oils, making it important

Ferri, B. *Complementary Health Approaches for Occupational Therapists* (pp. 43-47).
© 2021 Taylor & Francis Group.

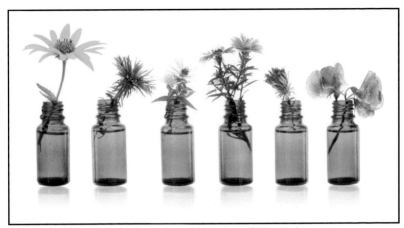

Figure 9-1. Oils are typically plant-based. MAXSHOT-PL/Shutterstock.com

to trust the source of the oils. When purchased from a verified manufacturer, essential oils are quite concentrated. This potency means everyone should research each essential oil before use and exercise caution to ensure the appropriate effect results (National Cancer Institute, 2018).

Using essential oils of impeccable quality is always recommended, so you must dilute the solution with some type of carrier oil. Carrier oils, such as almond, olive, avocado, jojoba, or coconut, will ensure the essential oil does not have a concentrated effect on the body. If you or a patient develop any skin reaction to essential oils, immediately apply any carrier oil to stop the reaction.

BENEFITS

Anecdotal evidence suggests aromatherapy is effective at improving and managing mood and other emotional symptoms. General research has shown mixed results. One study on the efficacy of general aromatherapy sessions showed no impact on physical symptoms, such as vital signs, pain, immunity, or wound healing. The same study showed lemon oil improved mood, while lavender had no effect on mood (Kiecolt-Glaser et al., 2008).

Another study determined that aromatherapy and massage on cancer patients improved comfort levels, stress and pain levels, muscle tension, lymphedema, quality of sleep, appetite levels, overall mood, and appetite. Participants also stated the oils brought an immediate sense of comfort, a slight boost to their mood, the sense of being cared for, and a connection to what they had previously thought of as a sickly body (Ho et al., 2017).

There are varying benefits associated with the use of each essential oil. For more information on common essential oils, refer to Basics of Aromatherapy.

CONTRAINDICATIONS, PRECAUTIONS, AND SIDE EFFECTS

When applied externally, citrus oils (lemon, orange, or grapefruit) are contraindicated with sun exposure. Due to the photosensitivity of these oils, this interaction can cause skin sensitivity or even burns in most patients (whether they are sensitive to the oils or not).

External application of certain essential oils may cause an allergic reaction or skin sensitivity in some patients. It is important to do a skin test before ingesting or applying any essential oil to avoid causing any bodily reactions. Instructions for a skin test can be found in Basics of Aromatherapy. There is a risk of a reaction if any essential oil comes in contact with mucous membranes. Children should not ingest essential oils.

All essential oils should be stored with bottles closed tightly, as essential oils are volatile and will evaporate into the air quickly. All essential oils are flammable and should be stored in a safe place (National Cancer Institute, 2018).

CREDENTIALING

Aromatherapy is safe to perform after reviewing the associated risks and determining if they are applicable to your patients. While there is no license required to practice aromatherapy, there are training programs and accompanying certifications in aromatherapy. These are a good option for those who wish to practice aromatherapy with clients on a regular basis.

The National Association for Holistic Aromatherapy offers three levels of certifications, which all hold a prerequisite of basic training in anatomy and physiology. Level one certification consists of 50 hours of education and five case studies followed by a certification exam. Level two certification consists of 200 hours of education and 10 case studies followed by a certification exam. Level three certification consists of 300 hours of education and 20 case studies followed by a certification exam (National Association for Holistic Aromatherapy, 2017).

AROMATHERAPY AND OCCUPATIONAL THERAPY

Aromatherapy can be used as a preparatory activity for its mood-boosting benefits. The use of aromatherapy within standard patient care areas of hospitals and even some nursing homes may be prohibited due to the complexity of medical conditions and various sensitivities (e.g., patients with migraines, fluctuating blood pressures, and sensitivities to certain smells). However, some inhalation of essential oils can be done at the discretion of the therapist after assessing a patient's medical condition, willingness, and the intended benefit.

BASICS OF AROMATHERAPY

Peppermint oil has a fresh and alerting aroma. Peppermint is commonly added to cosmetics, such as soaps and lotions, and to such food items as breath mints and garnishes. Peppermint should not be applied to the throat or neck of children, nor should children inhale it. When ingested, peppermint oil may cause indigestion (National Center for Complementary and Integrative Health [NCCIH], 2016d). Some cursory studies indicate peppermint's effectiveness in those with irritable bowel syndrome, but there is not enough evidence to prove a direct link (Ford et al., 2008).

Lavender oil commonly has a flowery and calming aroma. Lavender is poisonous if ingested, so it should only be used topically or inhaled. Some lavender extracts can cause nausea, joint pain, or migraines so they should be used with caution (NCCIH, 2017a). There are mixed studies indicating lavender has some level of effectiveness on lowering stress, pain, and anxiety levels (Perry et al., 2012). However, there is not enough evidence to make a definitive link between each factor.

Orange oil typically has a bitter aroma and taste, which is why it is commonly referred to as bitter orange oil. There is not much research on the effectiveness of bitter orange oil, though some studies state its effectiveness in treating skin conditions, such as ringworm, athlete's foot, and other minor infections (Goldberg, 2000). Be mindful that ingesting bitter orange oil may cause fainting, heart attack, or stroke. This risk goes up when ingested with caffeine. Pregnant women should avoid ingesting bitter orange oil (NCCIH, 2016b).

Skin tests are an important way to ensure it is safe to use certain essential oils on a patient. To test for skin sensitivities, place a drop of undiluted oil (straight from the bottle) onto the least sensitive areas of skin. This can be on the soles of the feet or in the elbow crease. Wait 60 to 90 seconds, and then look for any reaction. If burning or skin redness occurs, this means the skin is experiencing sensitivity to the oil because it is too strong. If the skin begins to itch significantly, this means there is an allergic reaction. In the event of either reaction, immediately apply a carrier oil, such as almond, olive, avocado, jojoba, or coconut, to neutralize the effect of the essential oil.

The best place for a therapist to experiment with any essential oils is in an outpatient clinic or private practice setting. These settings typically have closed off areas, allowing less chance of the aromas affecting other patients with potential sensitivities.

An occupational therapist can train patients in the use of aromatherapy within their self-care routine or as a way to calm the mind to prepare for therapy. Patients should always be educated on the usage instructions along with potential benefits and risks associated with each essential oil. Recommending patients purchase reliable brands to ensure above-average quality is also good practice.

See Basics of Aromatherapy for an overview of common essential oils.

CONSIDERATIONS FOR PRACTICE

Therapists who use aromatherapy on patients should determine the specific symptom that they are targeting in order to identify what aromas would be most beneficial. Some therapists may choose to use certain essential oils with patients who demonstrate low registration of sensory input. However, therapists should especially be cautious in these situations, since experimenting with a variety of different oils may be less therapeutic than one oil, two oils, or a proportionate blend of oils. Before using any type of aromatherapy, therapists must individually assess each patient regarding their sensitivities to smells. Patients and therapists ideally should only use oils in a private, well-ventilated area to prevent triggering nearby individuals who may have sensitivities or a history of migraines.

Therapists may write aromatherapy-related goals in some of the following areas:

- Managing emotions, such as sadness, anger, or irritability
- Improving independence in the use of relaxation techniques
- Promoting sleep hygiene
- Increasing health management skills

CHAPTER 10

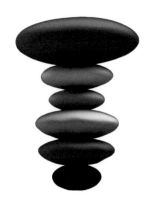

Art Therapy

Art therapy, sometimes referred to as *mindfulness-based art therapy*, is a modality using many forms of artwork to allow patients to engage in creative expression. This should not be confused with arts therapies, an umbrella term used to describe any of the modes of creative art expression, including music therapy, literature therapy, and dance therapy.

Art therapy allows for a different form of communication with oneself, their perceived reality, and those around them. Expression can be of internal conflicts, emotions, or general psychological status, and this method can assist an individual in moving toward emotional healing (Eum & Yim, 2015). Art therapy can be practiced through painting, the use of textiles, collage, carvings, pottery, card-making, claywork, drawing, sculpting, doodling, and finger painting (American Art Therapy Association, 2013) (Figure 10-1).

Ferri, B. *Complementary Health Approaches for Occupational Therapists* (pp. 49-52). © 2021 Taylor & Francis Group.

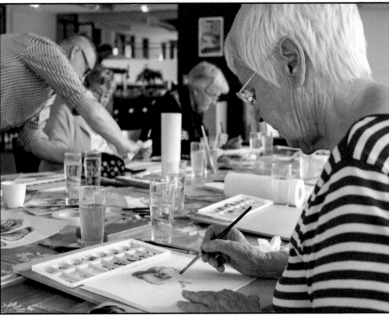

Figure 10-1. Art therapy can assume many forms, from painting to sculpting. belushi/ Shutterstock.com

BENEFITS

The American Art Therapy Association states that art therapy can help remedy emotional conflicts, promote self-awareness, regulate behavior, and mitigate the presence of addictions. Art therapy can also help to decrease anxiety, along with improve social skills, reality orientation, and self-esteem (2013).

Research shows that art therapy has improved communication between pediatric cancer patients, their family members, and health care providers (Aguilar, 2017). In dementia patients, art therapy has been shown to improve attention, lessen neuropsychiatric symptoms, improve social behavior, and enhance self-esteem (Chancellor et al., 2014). Research also shows a decrease in symptoms of depression and anxiety in patients who have experienced a stroke (Eum & Yim, 2015).

Due to its ability to improve behavioral and cognitive impairments, art therapy is typically indicated in a mental health population, with specific use for individuals with psychosis or a history of trauma.

Contraindications, Precautions, and Side Effects

Precautions of art therapy include risk of exploitation if an individual's personal artwork is shown in a public forum without their consent. When working with patients who have a history of trauma, there is the potential for the patient to relive such moments and cause an increase in psychiatric symptoms or a temporary setback in progress. There is the potential for this to happen whether the professional guiding the art therapy intends so or not. This can typically be avoided by receiving the appropriate training to gain an understanding of how to elicit emotion without causing a negative event.

Art therapy is contraindicated for individuals with severe psychiatric or cognitive deficits, as this may elicit too many suppressed emotions to serve the patient any benefit (Davis, 2017). Additionally, art therapy is contraindicated in patients with physical disabilities severe enough to impair the ability to manipulate artistic utensils.

Credentialing

A master's degree in art therapy is required to practice any part of art therapy. Education requirements consist of 100 hours of practical experience, along with 600 hours of supervised internships. Upon completion of these educational requirements from an approved and accredited art therapy program, individuals will be able to obtain certification as a registered art therapist. There are undergraduate programs in art therapy and, while these may prepare an individual prior to beginning a master's level program, these alone do not fulfill the requirement for certification (American Art Therapy Association, 2013).

Art Therapy and Occupational Therapy

As mentioned earlier, a master's degree in art therapy is required to practice art therapy with patients. However, occupational therapists can use art activities as part of therapy, with the intention of and focus on occupational therapy's treatment areas, including attention, memory, social interactions, leisure, upper extremity function, etc. To remain within occupational therapy's scope of practice, documentation should make no mention of art therapy unless the provider is a registered art therapist. As with all therapeutic and preparatory activities, each session should connect back to functional performance.

However, if an occupational therapist also holds a master's degree and certification in art therapy, they are able to combine the two practices to expand the range of services provided to patients. A practitioner who is both an occupational therapist and an art therapist would be able to effectively address the psychosocial and physical deficits of a patient in a treatment session. Art therapy may be best practiced individually; however, certain art-based activities can be used as a group activity to facilitate appropriate social interactions and the following of directions. Art activities can be performed at hospitals, nursing homes, outpatient settings, mental health settings, and school-based settings depending on supplies and facility space available.

CONSIDERATIONS FOR PRACTICE

Due to the risks associated with an unqualified professional providing art therapy to patients, therapists must implement this modality carefully and thoughtfully. Occupational therapists who wish to incorporate art into treatment can use a variety of mediums to prepare patients for other activities or to establish art as a hobby and healthy stress management tool. Therapists who use any kind of art must first assess a patient's safety awareness, cognition, and physical abilities as they pertain to the use of certain drawing utensils. If the therapist wants their patient to complete the art project while seated, patients should have access to an ergonomic setup with enough space to complete their task. Regardless of the art activity, patients should use materials that are appropriate for their abilities (e.g., a paintbrush with a built-up handle for someone who has arthritis in their fingers). Therapists can choose whether patients need a semiprivate area or not based on whether they think the patient would benefit from a group art activity or a secluded area where they can share personal stories related to their art.

Therapists may write art therapy–related goals in some of the following areas:

- Improving relaxation
- Establishing productive leisure
- Regulating behaviors
- Sequencing activity steps
- Strengthening seated or standing activity tolerance
- Planning and appropriately using tools
- Increasing gross range of motion of the shoulder, elbow, or wrist
- Improving fine motor strength, motion, and coordination
- Enhancing core strength, stability, and head/neck control

Chapter 11

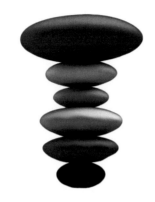

Auriculotherapy

Auriculotherapy is a modality in Chinese medicine that involves acupuncture of the ear (Figure 11-1). The Chinese believe the ear is reflective of the entire body, meaning specific points on the external ear represent organs, bones, muscles, and other bodily structures. This is similar to the premise of acupuncture, where each point targets a certain part of the body thought to have weakness.

Auriculotherapy is not used as a method of diagnosis; it is a technique associated with Traditional Chinese Medicine. A practitioner of Traditional Chinese Medicine may evaluate and determine the need for auriculotherapy according to an individual's symptoms and presentation.

Benefits

The benefits of auriculotherapy are similar to those of acupuncture, described in Chapter 6. Auriculotherapy has been proven to improve pain control and decrease the duration of labor in pregnant women (Mafetoni & Shimo, 2016). Additionally, short-term decreases in smoking habits

Ferri, B. *Complementary Health Approaches for Occupational Therapists* (pp. 53-56).
© 2021 Taylor & Francis Group.

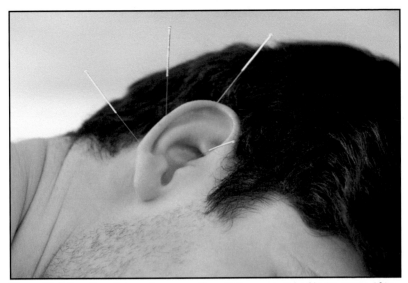

Figure 11-1. Specific points on the ear are thought to represent bodily structures. Africa Studio/Shutterstock.com

were noted in smokers who received auriculotherapy, with no reports of long-term benefits (Di et al., 2014).

Eight weeks of auriculotherapy sessions have also been noted to lessen the short-term recurrence of seizures in those with epilepsy (Rong et al., 2014). Research has also shown auriculotherapy can be used to increase subjective sleep recovery in those with insomnia. After 6 weeks of auriculotherapy sessions, individuals also had short-term reports of less difficulty waking up in the morning (Sjoling et al., 2008).

When older individuals with dementia received 3 months of auriculotherapy, researchers noted a decrease in challenging behaviors and sleep disturbances along with an increase in functional participation (Rodriguez-Mansilla et al., 2013).

CONTRAINDICATIONS, PRECAUTIONS, AND SIDE EFFECTS

The smaller risks associated with acupuncture also apply to the practice of auriculotherapy. Risks of acupuncture, such as collapsed lungs, are not present due to the acupuncture being performed on a much smaller scale. Additional risks associated with auriculotherapy are minor bleeding, fatigue, pain in the ear, dizziness, and temporary changes to skin on the ear (Tan et al., 2014).

Similar to acupuncture, auriculotherapy is contraindicated in patients with impaired blood clotting, weakened immune systems, pacemakers, and abnormal or artificial heart valves. These patients should not receive auriculotherapy due to the risk of infection (De Groot, 2001).

CREDENTIALING

Auriculotherapy cannot be practiced in any form without a certification and accompanying training. The Auriculotherapy Certification Institute states you must complete an educational program in order to qualify for certification (2014). Those interested must also complete 20 auriculotherapy case studies and pass a certification exam.

AURICULOTHERAPY AND OCCUPATIONAL THERAPY

As mentioned earlier, all forms of auriculotherapy can only be practiced with a certification in auriculotherapy. For those occupational therapy practitioners who possess this certification, the main area to use this modality would likely be private practice.

Hospitals, nursing homes, and other traditional therapy settings have restrictions relative to safety, location, complexity of patient medical conditions, and methods of service delivery. While auriculotherapy is more localized than acupuncture, which works on larger parts of the body, it remains difficult to implement outside of a private practice.

Occupational therapists who carry certification in auriculotherapy can combine it with other modalities that are geared toward the needs of their patients. Based on the populations that benefit from auriculotherapy, areas for occupational therapy treatment may include lifestyle redesign, nutritional recommendations, health and wellness consulting, symptom management, sleep hygiene, and more.

CONSIDERATIONS FOR PRACTICE

Auriculotherapy requires therapists to have an ample supply of single-use, sterile needles for each patient session. While this modality does not require the privacy that acupuncture does, therapists should find a quiet, semiprivate space to allow for enough concentration to perform auriculotherapy. Patients who are unfamiliar with or nervous about the use of needles for auriculotherapy should have additional amenities, such as soothing music, calming aromas, and comfortable blankets. Patients should receive written or verbal education on the risks of this modality and the benefits that they should experience. Therapists must provide individuals with continual instruction to ensure that their muscles are not tense throughout the process.

Therapists may write auriculotherapy-related goals in some of the following areas:

- Adhering to planned and scheduled auriculotherapy sessions to improve health management skills
- Lowering pain levels
- Tracking symptoms before and after auriculotherapy sessions
- Understanding the risks and intended benefits of auriculotherapy
- Increasing education regarding the mind-body connection
- Developing and maintaining a routine to improve sleep hygiene, quality, and quantity

CHAPTER 12

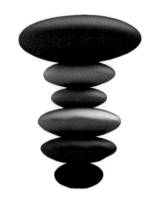

Bach Flower Essences

Bach Flower Essences, also known as *Bach Flower Remedies*, are a homeopathic modality developed by Dr. Edward Bach to address his idea of illness: Disharmony between body and mind. Bach believed illness was the external expression of poor emotional states. He experimented with liquid extracts from varying flowers and plants to find remedies for each negative emotional state (Figure 12-1). These extracts were mixed with equal parts brandy to formulate the final product.

Bach discovered 38 flower remedies to address each ailment. While more have been derived since the time of Bach in the early 1900s, they are not his original findings nor are they branded an original Bach Flower Essence.

There is also a line of products intended to alleviate emotional symptoms in animals, with specific guidelines for usage. Bach Flower Essences can be ingested, applied locally to areas of discomfort, or applied to acupressure points for a more systemic effect (Bach, 2019). A full list of the original Bach Flower Essences can be found in Basics of Bach Flower Essences.

Ferri, B. *Complementary Health Approaches for Occupational Therapists* (pp. 57-62). © 2021 Taylor & Francis Group.

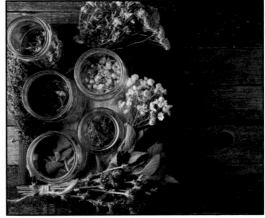

Figure 12-1. Bach used extracts from flowers and plants to alleviate distressing emotions. AkaciaArt/Shutterstock.com

BENEFITS

There is little research supporting the effectiveness of Bach Flower Essences. It is especially difficult to track its use due to the range of emotional symptoms each essence claims to remedy. A single-subject case report showed one postmenopausal woman experienced an improvement in objective sleep quality and sleep perception after taking a mix of Bach remedies for 4 months (Siegler et al., 2017). When applied locally, Bach Flower Essences have also proven effective in lessening pain and numbness in those with mild to moderate carpal tunnel syndrome (Rivas-Suarez et al., 2017).

A study showed that spirituality had a positive impact on the effectiveness of Bach Flower Essences in a sample population (Hyland et al., 2006). If you will recall, the main tenets of homeopathy are "like heals like" and "less is more," making room for an external force to fill in the gaps of physical intervention.

CONTRAINDICATIONS, PRECAUTIONS, AND SIDE EFFECTS

There are no known risks associated with taking Bach Flower Essences. Due to the 100% natural composition of the original remedies, fluctuations in dosage have no negative effect on the individual. Taking an entire bottle of the remedies, for example, is purported to have no adverse side effects. Children of any age and pregnant women can use Bach Flower Essences. Experimentation with the different remedies is not harmful. If someone takes a remedy for a negative emotion that is not present, there will be neither a positive nor a negative effect (Bach, 2019).

BASICS OF BACH FLOWER ESSENCES

Agrimony: For those who hide unhappiness through use of drugs and alcohol. These individuals use humor to mask their anxiety. Also for insomniacs.

Aspen: For those with vague fears of an unknown source and a terror regarding the possibility of something dreadful happening.

Beech: For those who are intolerant of the flaws in themselves and others. They have difficulty feeling compassion for others in their growing process.

Centaury: For those who cannot say no when imposed upon and overwork themselves to help others. They are passive and constantly lack energy.

Cerato: For those who lack the confidence to be firm in their own decisions. For those who always need advice from others and never trust their own wisdom.

Cherry Plum: For those who fear they will lose control, impulsively explode with anger, and have abusive tendencies. For those who feel about to simply break down.

Chestnut Bud: For those who take a long time to learn lessons of life. For those who keep repeating mistakes and cannot learn from past experiences.

Chicory: For those who are possessive, over-protective, and critical of others. They are constantly manipulating and controlling loved ones while self-pitying.

Clematis: For those who constantly daydream and cannot focus on the present. For the quiet and accident-prone who are unhappy and always live in the future.

Crab Apple: For those who feel the need to constantly clean themselves or their surroundings. They are anxious to be free from poor self-image or what poisons them.

Elm: For those who feel overwhelmed and depressed, with too much to do and no time for it all. The task undertaken is too difficult.

Gentian: For those who are easily discouraged by small setbacks. They are often depressed due to the happenings of daily life.

Gorse: For those who are constantly filled with hopelessness and despair that nothing more can fix them. They may try things to help but maintain their pessimistic state.

Heather: For those who are demanding of attention from everyone and are very talkative regarding their problems. They dislike being alone for any period.

(continued)

Basics of Bach Flower Essences (Continued)

Holly: For those with constant jealousy, suspicion, hatred, and aggression toward others. They are constantly suffering with seemingly no cause for unhappiness.

Honeysuckle: For those with homesickness who constantly live in the past. They expect no good to come of the future, as nothing compares to their past.

Hornbeam: For those who are weary and tire easily while doubting their abilities. They constantly feel they need more strength for any task. Burden of life is too heavy.

Impatiens: For those who are quick to action and thought, always irritated and nervous. They may be fidgety and accident-prone, wanting to work alone at own pace.

Larch: For those who lack confidence and feel inferior. They always expect failure, so they do not try or they make poor attempts to succeed.

Mimulus: For those who fear illness, pain, accident, poverty, misfortune, and being alone. They quietly dread this and are also shy about personal phobias.

Mustard: For those who feel deeply depressed for no reason, with no joy in their lives. Almost impossible to bring about any happiness.

Oak: For those who are exhausted and overworked. They blame themselves if they cannot work for any reason. They are overachievers in everything.

Olive: For those who lack the energy to make effort in anything. Daily life is too difficult for them.

Pine: For those who experience guilt and are constantly ashamed and apologetic. They always feel undeserving or unworthy of things they receive.

Red Chestnut: For those who are constantly worried for themselves and others. They are overly concerned with things that do not pertain to them.

Rock Rose: For those who experience freezing in the presence of terror. Good for after nightmares when they cannot reconnect with real life.

Rock Water: For those who set too high standards for themselves and sacrifice all pleasures that do not fit their perceived image. They enjoy being the martyr.

Scleranthus: For those who are indecisive and quiet. They choose not to speak of their difficulties with others. They are always uncertain to the point of dizziness at times.

(continued)

BASICS OF BACH FLOWER ESSENCES (CONTINUED)

Star of Bethlehem: For those under great distress, with a history of trauma. Good for those who refuse to be comforted from shock after an accident or death.

Sweet Chestnut: For those with extreme despair and unbearable anguish. When it seems there is nothing but destruction to face and intense sorrow to feel.

Vervain: For those who are overly enthusiastic, hyperactive, and high-strung. They wish to impose their views on everyone and are strong-willed.

Vine: For those who are very aggressive but capable and gifted. They are inflexible and certain of their own success and abilities.

Walnut: For those who cannot let go of the past. They fulfill all their strict ideals in life, but fall victim to temptations making them stray from their ideals.

Water Violet: For those who are proud but aloof and lonely. They are often clever and talented, but choose to be antisocial, condescending, and detached.

White Chestnut: For those who repeat unwanted thoughts and struggle to concentrate. They experience insomnia and mental torture from this.

Wild Oat: For those who have ambitions but lack clarity in decisions and cannot choose an occupation. This causes delay, dissatisfaction, and regret.

Wild Rose: For those who are apathetic and resigned to whatever happens in life. They use no effort to improve situations, lacking motivation and ambition.

Willow: For those who feel short-changed in response to hardships. They pity themselves and are sulky, irritable, and blame everything else for their situation (Bach, 2019).

Due to the absence of risks associated with Bach Flower Essences, there are no contraindications. As mentioned earlier, the impact of spirituality seems to influence how the remedies work. Therefore, it makes sense to say those who do not believe the remedies will work are likely to experience no emotional changes.

CREDENTIALING

No credentials are needed to use Bach Flower Essences in practice. A licensed health care professional or someone with no health care training can make recommendations for Bach Flower Essences.

For those interested in receiving training on Bach Flower Essences and their usage to improve emotional states, there is a three-level training program available to become a Bach Foundation registered practitioner through home study.

BACH FLOWER ESSENCES AND OCCUPATIONAL THERAPY

Due to the absence of risks and contraindications associated with Bach Flower Essences, use of the remedies can be incorporated into any health care setting. The remedies come in small bottles and can be easily applied or ingested.

For a practitioner who wishes to provide patient education on and experimentation with a variety of the 38 remedies, a private practice setting may be best. As with other complementary approaches, the use of Bach Flower Essences can be incorporated into a self-care routine as a preparatory method to relieve anxiety or other distressing emotions and improve participation in therapy.

CONSIDERATIONS FOR PRACTICE

Therapists who use Bach Flower Essences on patients should first determine the specific emotion or behavior that they are targeting in order to identify what flower essences would be most beneficial. Therapists should first assess if patients have sensitivities to certain smells or tastes. Most patients are comfortable simply placing a few drops of these flower essences on their tongue to elicit the desired response. However, patients who dislike the taste can mix it in water, juice, or herbal tea. Therapists must pinpoint the underlying emotion that is causing a patient distress in order to recommend the appropriate flower essence. Similar to aromatherapy, the flower essences may not be as effective if a patient is using multiple formulas at once. There are also blends of flower essences available from manufacturers who have combined essences that complement each other. In this case, patients can benefit from using multiple essences to address certain emotions or behaviors. Patients can use Bach Flower Essences in any setting, as this modality is discreet and does not require any additional tools or resources.

Therapists may write Bach Flower Essences–related goals in some of the following areas:
- Managing emotions, such as sadness, anger, or irritability
- Improving emotional awareness and intelligence
- Increasing the quality of relationships and social interactions
- Enhancing behavioral modification
- Promoting independence in the use of relaxation techniques
- Encouraging sleep hygiene and improved quality of sleep
- Using Bach Flower Essences daily as part of a self-care routine

CHAPTER 13

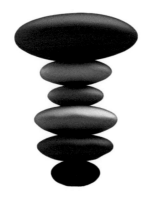

Biofeedback

Biofeedback is a modality that uses a device to monitor the functioning of the neuromuscular, respiratory, and cardiovascular systems. The user analyzes measurements of these vital signs in an attempt to regulate and control such functions for health improvement (Figure 13-1). Vital signs that can be monitored include heart rate variability, blood pressure, respirations, body temperature, brain waves, muscle contractions and tension, and sweat gland activity. Devices used to measure bodily activity include computer programs and wearable devices. Biofeedback is a noninvasive modality used to control certain health conditions or symptoms (Mayo Clinic, 2019).

BENEFITS

The Biofeedback Certification International Alliance (BCIA) states its effectiveness in addressing fecal and urinary incontinence, high blood pressure, temporomandibular joint disorder, peripheral nerve injury, and stroke (2019).

Ferri, B. *Complementary Health Approaches for Occupational Therapists* (pp. 63-67). © 2021 Taylor & Francis Group.

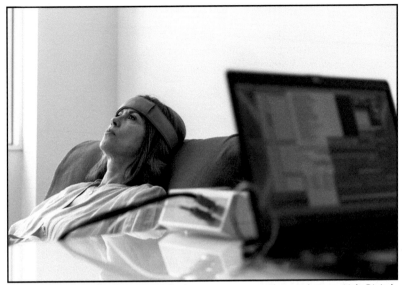

Figure 13-1. Biofeedback can track brain waves, among other vital signs. Malt Digital Agency/Shutterstock.com

Research has shown biofeedback is effective in lessening symptoms of depression, easing muscle tension, and improving mental clarity in those with chronic pain (Sielski et al., 2017). A biofeedback-based program was effective in improving the balance of children with autism spectrum disorder (Travers et al., 2018). Cardiovascular biofeedback has been deemed effective for individuals with high blood pressure, chronic heart failure, asthma, and fibromyalgia (Giggins et al., 2013).

While biofeedback has been reported effective in those with musculoskeletal issues, little research has been done in the area of sport performance. One study showed athletes who participated in biofeedback training demonstrated improved psychophysiological variables leading to improved sport performance (Jimenez-Morgan & Molina-Mora, 2017).

CONTRAINDICATIONS, PRECAUTIONS, AND SIDE EFFECTS

While biofeedback is a safe and noninvasive modality, it is contraindicated for use in those with heart arrhythmia. Monitoring devices can further interfere with abnormal heart rhythms, causing cardiac arrest. Those with certain skin conditions that impact adherence of electrodes to the skin should also not use biofeedback. This impacts a device's ability to measure vital signs. There are no recorded precautions or side effects of biofeedback.

BASICS OF BIOFEEDBACK

Breathing: Flexible bands are placed around the abdomen and chest to monitor breathing pattern and rate of respiration. This is commonly used to perform biofeedback on individuals with asthma, chronic obstructive pulmonary disease, hypertension, and other cardiopulmonary disorders.

Heart rate variability: Sensors are placed on the chest, earlobe, and finger to measure time between each heartbeat. This is commonly used to perform biofeedback on individuals with anxiety, asthma, depression, hypertension, post-traumatic stress disorder, pre-eclampsia, and other cardiovascular disorders.

Muscle tension: Also known as *electromyography*, muscle tension measures electrical activity using sensors over skeletal muscles. This is commonly used to perform biofeedback on individuals with anxiety, asthma, cerebral palsy, fecal and urinary incontinence, migraines, hypertension, low back pain, pelvic pain, temporomandibular joint disorder, peripheral nerve injury, stroke, and other musculoskeletal or neurological disorders.

Sweat gland activity: Also known as *electrodermal activity*, sweat gland activity is measured using sensors placed on the fingers and palm. These sensors measure changes in skin moisture. This is commonly used to perform biofeedback on individuals with anxiety, excessive sweating, and hypertension.

Temperature: Sensors are placed on the hands and feet to measure blood flow to the skin. This is commonly used to perform biofeedback on individuals with hypertension, Raynaud's disease, edema, and vascular headaches (BCIA, 2019) (Figure 13-2).

CREDENTIALING

In order to practice biofeedback, a certification is recommended but not required. No license is available for biofeedback. BCIA requires individuals seeking a full certification in biofeedback to hold a current license and bachelor's degree in physical therapy or nursing.

Full entry-level certification in biofeedback requires 42 hours of didactic training followed by 10 sessions of self-regulation, 50 patient sessions, and 10 case studies. Individuals can also be certified by prior experience if they have documented an advanced number of patient hours over the past 5 years.

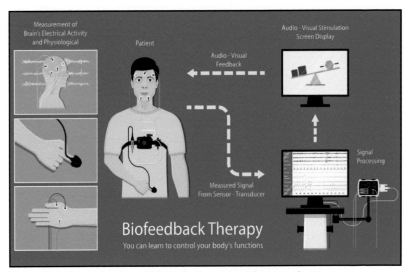

Figure 13-2. The mechanisms of biofeedback. rumruay/Shutterstock.com

These certification processes are different; however, both will allow providers the same capabilities. There is also the option for a technician certification that will only allow the practitioner to practice biofeedback within the scope of practice of their certified supervisor (BCIA, 2019).

BIOFEEDBACK AND OCCUPATIONAL THERAPY

Therapists trained in its use can incorporate biofeedback into any setting. This can be used as a preparatory activity to calm individuals with psychiatric disorders, stimulate muscle activity in the neurologically impaired, relieve muscle tension in those with musculoskeletal symptoms, and more. The use of biofeedback can prepare a range of individuals for better engagement in functional tasks. Some therapists may find it fitting to recommend a home monitoring device for patients who find especially good success with biofeedback and wish to continue regular use of this modality.

CONSIDERATIONS FOR PRACTICE

Therapists who perform biofeedback on patients must have a working, fully inspected biofeedback machine along with attachments to measure brain waves and other vital signs. Because biofeedback measures a patient's vital signs and the body's stress response, it is important to take these measurements in a private, quiet area to allow the machine to receive an accurate reading. Therapists can later work with patients to develop daily plans and relaxation techniques in any setting. The biofeedback machine must be properly stored along with all of its attachments, so therapists must have access to a temperature-controlled area for safekeeping. Therapists need training on how to use the biofeedback machine, but they should not need any other special preparation to use biofeedback on patients once they have the credentials to do so.

Therapists may write biofeedback-related goals in some of the following areas:

- Regulating behaviors
- Enhancing relaxation
- Practicing mindfulness
- Improving body awareness
- Recognizing unhealthy behaviors
- Developing plans to use healthy, productive routines and habits
- Understanding the mind-body connection and how it pertains to their life

CHAPTER 14

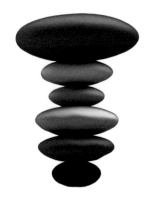

Chiropractic Manipulation

Chiropractic manipulation, also known as *chiropractic adjustment*, is performed using hands (manual techniques) or small instruments (Figure 14-1). Whether or not an instrument is used, a controlled but sudden force applied to the spine is needed to improve mobility and overall bodily function. Vertebral misalignment is thought to have an impact on other portions of the body, causing pain, swelling, nerve sensitivities, and other symptoms.

Even if someone's presentation matches the aforementioned symptoms, this does not guarantee an individual will respond to manipulation through chiropractic adjustment. This is typically because not every individual's pain and nerve involvement is the result of vertebral misalignment.

While manipulation is one of the main modalities provided by chiropractors, chiropractic care can consist of applied heat, ice, electrical stimulation, strengthening exercises, lifestyle recommendations, and dietary supplements (National Center for Complementary and Integrative Health [NCCIH], 2012).

Ferri, B. *Complementary Health Approaches for Occupational Therapists* (pp. 69-72). © 2021 Taylor & Francis Group.

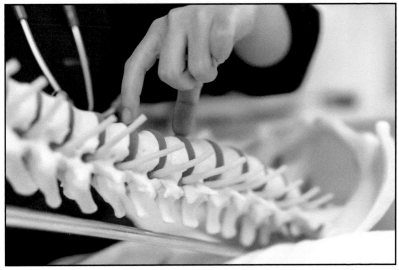

Figure 14-1. Chiropractic adjustments manipulate the spine. nuiza11/Shutterstock.com

BENEFITS

Chiropractic adjustments can benefit individuals with lower back pain, neck pain, migraines, upper extremity joint conditions, and whiplash (NCCIH, 2012). Research on spinal manipulation and other chiropractic alignments has mainly shown an improvement in lower back pain. Studies have shown, when compared to conventional treatment protocols, chiropractic manipulation was equally as effective or more effective in reducing acute pain (Bialosky et al., 2009).

CONTRAINDICATIONS, PRECAUTIONS, AND SIDE EFFECTS

The side effects associated with chiropractic manipulation are brief headaches, fatigue, or discomfort to the area manipulated. Precautions include risk of developing or worsening a herniated disc, spinal nerve compression, or stroke (after manipulation of the neck).

Chiropractic manipulation is contraindicated for individuals with severe osteoporosis, nerve sensitivity or sensation changes in the extremities, spinal cancer, and bone abnormalities in the spine or neck. Chiropractic manipulation is also contraindicated for individuals who are at risk for a stroke (Mayo Clinic, 2018; NCCIH, 2013a).

CREDENTIALING

Occupational therapists are able to perform manual techniques on patients according to their scope of practice or, if applicable, specialty certification or training. In order to perform chiropractic manipulation of the spine on patients, an individual must hold a license to practice chiropractic care or chiropractic medicine. Practitioners of chiropractic care are also called doctors of chiropractic medicine.

The American Chiropractic Association states that training for chiropractors consists of a 4-year clinical doctoral degree with a minimum of 4,200 hours of education and internships (2019). However, it is important to remember that practitioners in the field of chiropractic care have not completed medical school nor are they medical doctors.

CHIROPRACTIC MANIPULATION AND OCCUPATIONAL THERAPY

As mentioned earlier, a doctoral degree and accompanying license to practice chiropractic medicine are required to incorporate chiropractic manipulation into occupational therapy treatment. This can be done in any setting; however, those therapists who possess training and licensure in both fields would likely be best suited in private practice to expand the availability of services provided.

For those therapists who have patients receiving chiropractic care from a practitioner while receiving occupational therapy services, it is appropriate to educate patients on how to safely exercise to complement these services.

CONSIDERATIONS FOR PRACTICE

Therapists trained in the use of chiropractic manipulation should have a private area where patients can comfortably remove articles of clothing, as needed according to the body part(s) that are targeted. Some therapists may use tools or instruments to assist them in manipulating certain larger parts of a patient's body, such as muscles in the leg or back. Therapists should always determine a patient's current levels of pain, stiffness, and other symptoms before manipulating. Patients should receive written or verbal education on the risks of this modality and the benefits that they should experience. Therapists must provide individuals with continual instruction to ensure that patients maintain appropriate body positions and muscle relaxation throughout the process. Patients should also be able to verbalize pain or discomfort throughout the process, if this does occur. Most therapists will develop a specific plan regarding what body part to manipulate but can alter the plan if patients present with varied symptoms before their session.

Therapists may write chiropractic-related goals in some of the following areas:

- Lowering pain levels
- Increasing range of motion to the neck, shoulder, or other body parts
- Improving mobility and functional performance
- Enhancing postural symmetry and quality of movement
- Tracking symptoms before and after manipulation
- Using ergonomic posture and techniques along with joint protection strategies to maintain proper body alignment

CHAPTER 15

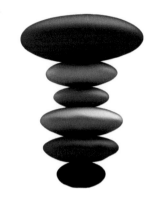

Chromotherapy

Chromotherapy, also known as *color therapy*, uses the healing effects of colors in the visible spectrum to relieve certain symptoms or discomfort. By using the innate energies or vibrations that each color holds, chromotherapy aims to increase an individual's vibrational frequencies. The specific vibrations associated with each color are thought to have an impact on an individual's physical and mental health.

Each color used in traditional chromotherapy is associated with one of the seven chakras of the body (Figure 15-1). The use of these specific colors may heal imbalances to the chakras, as they are closely related.

These vibrational changes are promoted through lights, lasers, clothing, food, crystals, gemstones, glass, water, and plants that are colored according to an individual's specific conditions or ailments. Receiving care through a color therapist involves more than simply exposing someone to colored objects. However, individuals can incorporate the addition of healing colors in their daily lives for an added boost (Przybyla, 2018).

Ferri, B. *Complementary Health Approaches for Occupational Therapists* (pp. 73-77). © 2021 Taylor & Francis Group.

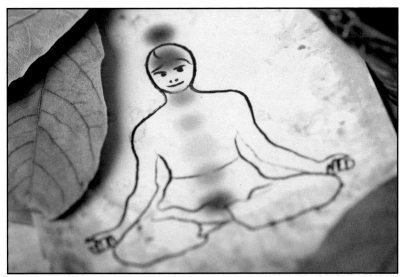

Figure 15-1. Color therapy is based off the seven chakras of the body. Monika Wisniewska/ Shutterstock.com

BENEFITS

Anecdotal evidence suggests the color red can stimulate blood and lymph flow, while the color orange can heal the thyroid gland, and the color yellow can stimulate cognitive function. Further anecdotal evidence states green can heal heart conditions, blue can ease inflammation, and purple can stimulate the immune system and improve insomnia. However, there is a scarcity of research proving the efficacy of chromotherapy for these purposes.

There are historical recordings stating the use of colors to encourage physical healing. Around 980 A.D., the color red was used to move the blood, the colors blue and white were used to cool the blood, and the color yellow was used to reduce pain and swelling. Research by Robert Gerard in the 1950s focused on the review of the physiological effects of color. He found warm colors were effective in increasing the arousal and attentiveness of those with depression or neurological disorders. Warm colors also served to increase muscle tone and blood pressure in individuals with hypertension, while increasing respirations, blinking, and activating the autonomic nervous system (Gerard, 1958).

Cooler colors were found to calm those with anxiety and acted as a natural tranquilizer. These same cool colors lowered blood pressure, decreased blinking, calmed muscle spasms, and helped those with insomnia (Yousuf Azeemi & Mohsin-Raza, 2005). Specific research related to colored light therapy will be detailed in a later chapter.

BASICS OF CHROMOTHERAPY

Blue: Represents loving, nurturing, and support. Also meant to foster love, relationships, and spirituality. Blue typically attracts those who are healers, teachers, and counselors.

Green: Represents power and intelligence. Also extremely bright, standing for those with a strong will and quick thinking. Green typically attracts those drawn to money, power, and business.

Indigo: Represents new energy, peace, and harmony. Also stands for honesty, awareness, and independence. Indigo typically attracts those who are fearless and those with psychic abilities.

Lavender: Represents fantasy, enchantment, and spiritual beings. Lavender typically attracts dreamers, wanderers, and those who feel reality is too harsh.

Magenta: Represents nonconformity and rebellion. Also stands for shocking others and living on their own path. Magenta typically attracts loners and those who desire freedom.

Orange: Represents thrill seeking and feeling alive. Also stands for risk and high-stakes activities. Orange typically attracts those who are cunning and thrive off excitement.

Red: Represents abstract thinking and strength. Also stands for living in the here and now with courage and self-confidence. Red typically attracts those who express themselves through sensuality and their physical bodies.

Violet: Represents inspiration, safety, and improvement. Also stands for charisma and quality of life. Violet typically attracts those who are visionaries, leaders, and those who wish to save the planet.

Yellow: Represents fun loving, energy, spontaneity, and childlike traits. Also stands for optimism, joy, and sensitivity. Yellow typically attracts those who are shy or those who are outgoing (Przybyla, 2018).

CONTRAINDICATIONS, PRECAUTIONS, AND SIDE EFFECTS

Due to the use of nonmedical devices or formulas, the noninvasive methods of chromotherapy (e.g., gemstones, crystals, water, food) do not pose any risks to patients.

One area of chromotherapy focuses on light therapy, and this area may have risks associated if used on medically complex patients. Precautions involving colored light therapy include vision changes if completed improperly. Chromotherapy involving the use of colored lights is contraindicated for patients who are prone to seizures or who have vision deficits.

CREDENTIALING

No license or certifications are required to practice chromotherapy; however, training and certification is available to those who wish to pursue it. This training is not limited to health care professionals, as there are no anatomy- or kinesiology-related courses required to learn chromotherapy. Certifications can be sought online, but individuals may practice the basics of chromotherapy in their personal lives or their health care practice without it.

CHROMOTHERAPY AND OCCUPATIONAL THERAPY

Occupational therapists can use chromotherapy in treatment by incorporating color principles as a preparatory method. Due to its ease of use and the ability for individuals to use it in their personal lives, clients can be educated to use more color to reap the emotional benefits associated with each color. The basics of chromotherapy can be found on the next page.

The principles of chromotherapy can be used on individual patients or in group therapy across hospitals, nursing homes, schools, outpatient clinics, and private practice settings. Patients can also be taught to incorporate the use of various colors within their self-care routine.

CONSIDERATIONS FOR PRACTICE

Therapists who use chromotherapy on patients should first identify if patients have certain tactile, visual, auditory, gustatory, or olfactory sensitivities or preferences. Chromotherapy may include the use of or exposure to lights, textures, smells, food, clothing, and other objects of various colors. Once a therapist has identified any stimulus that they should avoid, they can experiment with a range of different colors and observe the impact that each item has on a patient's mood and behaviors. Therapists can experiment with colors in a variety of therapy or community settings, such as parks, forests, nature trails, bodies of water, and more. Therapists can then work with patients to develop a plan for integrating the most beneficial and preferred colored objects into their daily routines. Therapists may use many informal tools, as color comes in the form of many objects. Some therapists may prefer to plan the use of some objects, while other therapists may opt to use impromptu tools that they discover with their patients during a session. Based on therapist judgment and patient preference, patients can participate in chromotherapy individually or in a group setting.

Therapists may write chromotherapy-related goals in some of the following areas:

- Enhancing behavioral modification
- Promoting independence in the use of relaxation techniques
- Using chromotherapy daily or as needed as part of a self-care routine
- Increasing awareness of personal preferences and responses to certain colors
- Improving a patient's ability to identify emotions and use them in a productive manner
- Encouraging creativity and self-expression when seeking out various colors in their daily lives during activities, such as writing or painting

CHAPTER 16

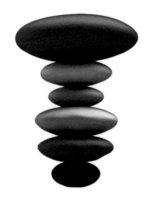

Craniosacral Therapy

Craniosacral therapy is a modality used to release muscle tension and joint restriction near the brain and spinal cord. This is meant to restore normal function by improving bodily processes (Jakel & Von Hauenschild, 2012). Similar to chiropractic manipulation, craniosacral therapy involves the use of manual techniques. However, rather than gross adjustments, craniosacral therapy uses light touch as a form of manipulation (Figure 16-1). Since light touch is local to the spinal cord and brain, tension alleviated serves to improve the flow of spinal fluid. This encourages the body's natural ability to heal itself of certain symptoms.

BENEFITS

Anecdotal evidence suggests craniosacral therapy is effective in addressing migraines, constipation, irritable bowel syndrome, insomnia, scoliosis, recurrent respiratory or ear infections, neck pain, fibromyalgia, temporomandibular joint disorder, whiplash, and mood disorders.

Ferri, B. *Complementary Health Approaches for Occupational Therapists* (pp. 79-82).
© 2021 Taylor & Francis Group.

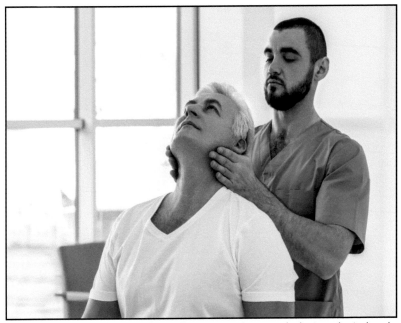

Figure 16-1. Light touch is thought to relieve pressure between the brain and spinal cord. Africa Studio/Shutterstock.com

However, there is a scarcity of research proving the efficacy of craniosacral therapy for use with these conditions.

When compared to classic massage, research shows individuals with low-back pain who received craniosacral therapy demonstrated decreased pain intensity and increased oxygen saturation. Additional benefits include an increase in systolic blood pressure along with increased blood levels of potassium and magnesium (Castro-Sanchez et al., 2016).

Research showed craniosacral therapy was effective in decreasing overall bodily pain and cervical pain, while increasing reaction time, short-term memory, cervical range of motion, and sleep quantity in males with postconcussion syndrome (Wetzler et al., 2017).

CONTRAINDICATIONS, PRECAUTIONS, AND SIDE EFFECTS

Precautions associated with craniosacral therapy include the risk of discomfort or even moderate pain to the area where therapy was performed. There have been some reports of individuals experiencing an aneurysm or head injury following craniosacral therapy; however, this was likely due to the underlying presence of an aneurysm or head injury.

Craniosacral therapy is contraindicated for patients with bleeding disorders, aneurysms, or those with a recent history of head injuries. These head injuries may include skull fractures, brain injuries, or any cranial bleeding (Gotter, 2017).

CREDENTIALING

No license is required to practice craniosacral therapy. There are certifications available for those who wish to practice this modality on patients. Most states will require those individuals who practice craniosacral therapy to also hold a license in a profession that involves the use of manual techniques, including doctors of chiropractic medicine, physical therapists, occupational therapists, and massage therapists. Possessing a license with a scope of practice, including manual therapies, lessens the liability on the individual, since there is no license protecting those who practice solely craniosacral therapy.

In order to enter a certification program for craniosacral therapy, a background in anatomy is required. Those with active health care licenses will fulfill this requirement. After completing two levels of educational content and 75 protocol sessions, an individual will need to pass the exam to receive a certification in craniosacral therapy. This will enable individuals to use the initials "CST" after their name (Upledger Institute International, 2019).

CRANIOSACRAL THERAPY AND OCCUPATIONAL THERAPY

Occupational therapists are able to complete manual therapies, including deep input and light touch, as part of their scope. Billed under manual techniques, this serves to decrease inflammation, increase body awareness, and improve motion in preparation for activity. While an occupational therapist is able to perform all aspects of touch therapy, the practitioner should not promote craniosacral therapy as a service they provide unless they possess the certification and experience to do so.

For those therapists trained in craniosacral, they can incorporate it into any practice setting where manual techniques would be. As with any intervention, a therapist should perform an evaluation and identify any contraindications before adding this modality to a treatment plan. Craniosacral therapy can be used to improve participation in a range of functional activities when completed during individual sessions with patients. This modality is best suited for outpatient clinics or private practice settings, as hospitalized patients often are not medically stable enough for craniosacral therapy.

CONSIDERATIONS FOR PRACTICE

While craniosacral therapy does not require therapists to use any tools or patients to remove any articles of clothing, patients would still benefit from a private area to ensure for their comfort. Patients may also benefit from additional amenities, such as soothing music, calming aromas, and comfortable blankets to promote a feeling of ease. Therapists should always determine a patient's current levels of pain, stiffness, and other physical or emotional symptomology before using this modality. Patients should receive written or verbal education on the risks of craniosacral therapy and the benefits they should experience. Therapists must provide individuals with continual instruction to ensure that patients maintain appropriate body positions and muscle relaxation throughout the process. Therapists must also inform patients to verbalize any discomfort throughout the process, if this does occur.

Therapists may write craniosacral therapy–related goals in some of the following areas:

- Lowering pain levels
- Increasing range of motion to the head, neck, shoulder, or other body parts
- Improving mobility and functional performance
- Enhancing postural symmetry and quality of movement
- Tracking symptoms before and after craniosacral therapy
- Using ergonomic posture and techniques along with joint protection strategies to maintain proper body alignment

CHAPTER 17

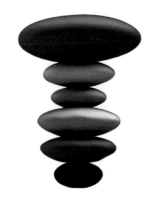

Cupping Therapy

Cupping therapy is a modality of Traditional Chinese Medicine that involves placement of round cups on parts of the body (Figure 17-1). In the traditional cupping process, cups are placed after a flammable mixture is added inside to produce a vacuum effect. Substances applied may include paper, herbs, or alcohol. Modern implementation of cupping may instead use a pump to create a vacuum effect.

Cups may be removed after 10 minutes, or they may be rapidly attached and removed from the body to produce the same effect. The latter version of cupping is often used with a skin emollient to produce a massage-like effect. The vacuum effect is intended to draw forward the skin underneath, increase blood flow to the local area, and increase the flow of energy, or *qi*. This movement of qi is thought to balance any weak areas of the body while remedying illnesses or injuries that may be present. Another form of cupping involves small punctures to the skin before applying the cups, causing what is intended to be a detoxifying effect by allowing blood to flow into the cups (Wong, 2019).

Ferri, B. *Complementary Health Approaches for Occupational Therapists* (pp. 83-86). © 2021 Taylor & Francis Group.

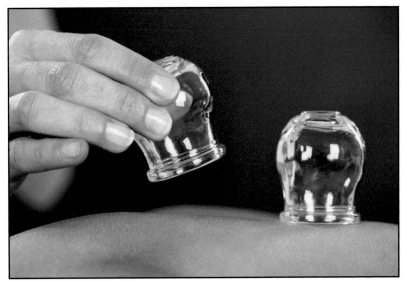

Figure 17-1. Cupping is often used in conjunction with massage therapy. Andrey_Popov/ Shutterstock.com

BENEFITS

Anecdotal evidence suggests that cupping therapy can assist with a range of joint pain, muscle pain, migraines, and sports injuries. However, there is minimal evidence supporting the effectiveness of cupping therapy.

Research shows cupping therapy is effective in decreasing pain levels and improving the perceived quality of life in patients with fibromyalgia (Lauche et al., 2016). Additional studies show cupping therapy assisted in decreasing pain levels of those with lower back pain (Wang et al., 2017).

Another study shows the efficacy of cupping therapy on decreasing pain, stiffness, and improving the overall physical function of individuals with osteoarthritis of the knee when combined with conventional treatments (Li et al., 2017). Research also suggests cupping therapy is beneficial in improving perceptions of pain and disability, increasing range of motion, and reducing creatine kinase in athletes (Bridgett et al., 2018).

CONTRAINDICATIONS, PRECAUTIONS, AND SIDE EFFECTS

Side effects associated with cupping include dizziness, increased sweating, changes in skin texture or pigmentation, nausea, swelling, blisters, burns, and pain or discomfort to the area where cupping was performed. Side effects related to the skin typically subside after several days or weeks; however, scarring has occurred in those with sensitive skin. Severe side effects include acquired hemophilia, anemia, and thrombocytopenia. Side effects associated with wet cupping, where the skin is punctured, include infection, scarring, and minor to moderate blood loss.

Cupping is contraindicated on areas with open wounds, fractures, injured arteries, veins, or lymph nodes, and inflamed or irritated skin. Cupping is also contraindicated in children, pregnant women, those who are taking blood thinners, older adults, and individuals with cancer, blood diseases, heart disease, or organ failure (Wong, 2019).

CREDENTIALING

Cupping is a modality commonly used by massage therapists who have completed training followed by subsequent certification and licensure. Those without a massage therapy credential can pursue training and certification in cupping therapy. There is currently no license available to practice cupping therapy.

The National Certification Board for Therapeutic Massage and Bodywork provides courses on cupping therapy with the option of specializing in cupping for those who complete the training. The International Cupping Therapy Association also provides certifications in contemporary cupping methods. These certifications have a prerequisite of anatomy courses along with training and work experience in manual therapy techniques. Certification requirements consist of an educational period followed by providing 24 patient sessions (International Cupping Therapy Association, n.d.).

CUPPING THERAPY AND OCCUPATIONAL THERAPY

Only certified and trained professionals can perform cupping therapy. Those who possess this certification can incorporate cupping into hospitals, nursing facilities, and outpatient clinics as part of their occupational therapy treatment. Cupping should be provided as a method to improve physical function in those patients who are deemed able to benefit from the modality. As with any intervention, a complete evaluation should be completed and contraindications should be ruled out prior to use of cupping therapy.

Cupping should be completed during individual sessions and can be used to encourage relaxation and physical benefits in patients. This modality can be incorporated into a regular self-care routine to enhance functional performance if patients wish to continue cupping on a regular basis.

CONSIDERATIONS FOR PRACTICE

Therapists trained in the use of cupping therapy should have a private area where patients can comfortably remove articles of clothing, as needed according to the body part(s) that are targeted.

Patients may also benefit from additional amenities, such as soothing music, calming aromas, and comfortable blankets to promote a feeling of ease. Therapists must determine a patient's current levels of pain, inflammation, or other symptomology before using cupping therapy. Therapists need access to enough sterile, safe cups along with emollient such as lotion or oils to use alongside the cups, if they choose. Therapists must ensure that patients do not have any allergies to certain ingredients before using lotions or oils. Patients should receive written or verbal education on the risks of this modality and the benefits they should experience. Patients should also be able to verbalize pain or discomfort throughout the process, if this does occur.

Therapists may write cupping therapy–related goals in some of the following areas:

- Encouraging relaxation
- Lowering pain levels
- Reducing inflammation
- Increasing range of motion to the head, neck, or shoulders
- Improving mobility and functional performance
- Enhancing postural symmetry and quality of movement
- Tracking symptoms before and after cupping therapy

CHAPTER 18

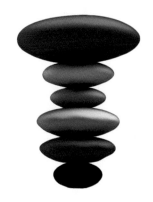

Electromagnetic Therapy

Electromagnetic therapy, also known as *magnetic therapy*, is a modality involving the application of low-frequency, time-varying electromagnetic fields via magnets to induce a current strong enough to activate tissue. This force intends to act on the varying levels of energy in electrical particles within the body. Current provided rebalances bodily energies of the epidermis, dermis, subcutaneous tissue, tendons, muscles, and bones to address various conditions (Figure 18-1). Practitioners use their clinical judgement to make frequency adjustments based on the organs targeted and session length (Weintraub, 2004).

There are several types of magnetic therapy that only practitioners can perform. Static or permanent magnetic field therapy is the application of one or several magnets and electrical current through a coil to the body. Other types are considered time-varying, including transcranial magnetic stimulation using 1 to 200 Hz, low-frequency electromagnetic fields using 50 to 60 Hz, pulsed radiofrequency fields using 12 to 42 MHz, and

Ferri, B. *Complementary Health Approaches
for Occupational Therapists* (pp. 87-90).
© 2021 Taylor & Francis Group.

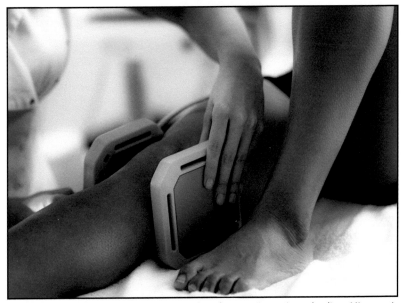

Figure 18-1. Low-frequency magnets are thought to activate tissue healing. Microgen/Shutterstock.com

millimeter waves using 30 to 100 GHz. Hospitals commonly use repetitive transcranial magnetic stimulation and high-frequency transcranial magnetic stimulation (De Loecker et al., 1990).

Pulsed electromagnetic fields (PEMF) are commonly recommended for home use. PEMF uses 5 to 300 Hz through magnets of specific shapes and quantities, along with varying amplitudes (Vadala et al., 2015). Licensed professionals can combine magnetic therapy with acupuncture by applying magnets to points that are similar to acupuncture points.

BENEFITS

Anecdotal evidence shows PEMF therapy can be helpful in addressing arthritis pain, wounds, insomnia, headaches, and pain related to fibromyalgia.

Current academic thoughts on the topic state electromagnetism can stop the progression of inflammation, while influencing genetic material to regenerate healthy tissue (Gordon, 2007). However, there is a lack of recent research proving its efficacy. One dated study using pulsed electromagnetic therapy on those with chronic neck pain showed a decrease in pain levels and an increase in range of motion (Foley-Nolan et al., 1990). Another dated study analyzed the benefit of PEMF on tendinitis of the rotator cuff, showing varying results of decreased pain after 8 weeks (Binder et al., 1984).

Growing trends have evolved using magnets in the form of bracelets, bandages, shoe insoles, or mattress inserts to elicit this same effect at home. However, scientific research does not support the efficacy of these trends.

CONTRAINDICATIONS, PRECAUTIONS, AND SIDE EFFECTS

Side effects of electromagnetic therapy may include nausea, dizziness, and generalized pain. Electromagnetic therapy is contraindicated in those who have pacemakers or insulin pumps, as the electrical current can interfere with these devices. Electromagnetic therapy is also contraindicated in pregnant women.

CREDENTIALING

There is no license to practice electromagnetic therapy. The American Association of Drugless Practitioners requires completion of a certification program to practice electromagnetic therapy. There are no prerequisites for certification, and an individual does not have to be a health care practitioner to receive this certification. Training is typically provided online with 20 hours of educational content and a certification exam at the end. Hands-on training is optional in the form of a one-day manual training course (Magna Wave, 2019).

ELECTROMAGNETIC THERAPY AND OCCUPATIONAL THERAPY

If therapists possess a certification in electromagnetic therapy, they can incorporate it into occupational therapy treatment as a preparatory method or manual technique. Depending on the patient's presenting problems, therapists can use this modality to decrease pain or increase movement to improve patient participation in the remainder of the therapy session. As with any modality, this should not be incorporated into therapy without first completing an evaluation and assessing possible contraindications.

Occupational therapists can use this modality during individual treatment sessions in hospitals, nursing homes, outpatient clinics, and private practice settings, if space and resources allow. This modality is likely best suited for outpatient clinics or private practice settings due to the space needed for this modality to be performed.

CONSIDERATIONS FOR PRACTICE

Therapists who perform electromagnetic therapy on patients must have a working, fully inspected device. Because electromagnetic therapy requires the use of low-level magnetic stimulation, patients should be in a private area for their own safety and the safety of others. Patients are typically best suited in a reclined position on a padded treatment table to encourage them to remain still, comfortable, and relaxed. All equipment must be properly stored, so therapists must have access to a temperature-controlled area for safekeeping. Therapists need training on how to use the necessary devices, but they should not need any other special preparation to use electromagnetic therapy on patients once they have the credentials to do so. Therapists should only use this modality after they have completed a thorough evaluation for the safety of their patients.

Therapists may write electromagnetic therapy–related goals in some of the following areas:

- Improving mobility and functional performance
- Enhancing postural symmetry and quality of movement
- Lowering pain levels
- Increasing range of motion to certain injured or affected joints
- Tracking symptoms before and after electromagnetic therapy
- Using ergonomic posture and techniques along with joint protection strategies to maintain proper body alignment

CHAPTER 19

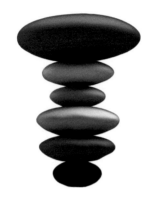

Emotional Freedom Techniques

Emotional Freedom Techniques (EFT) is a type of energy psychology used to balance the energies within the body. EFT is a simple combination of words and gestures used to lessen the intensity of negative memories. EFT can be used on negative memories as small as minor car accidents or as large as deeply traumatic events, such as witnessing a death. Many of us do not even realize the impact of negative memories from our past, but each one influences our lives in the present.

Though EFT focuses on emotions by working on negative memories, it can also be used to lessen the impact of physical ailments. Due to EFT's combination of words and gestures, it has often been called acupuncture without needles. This is because the gestures often involve an individual tapping on these meridian points within the body (Church, 2012) (Figure 19-1).

Ferri, B. *Complementary Health Approaches for Occupational Therapists* (pp. 91-95). © 2021 Taylor & Francis Group.

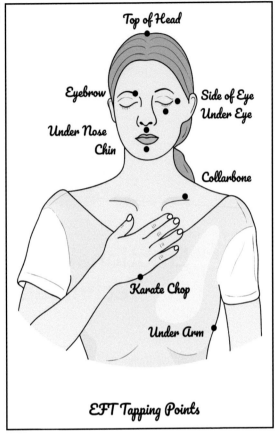

BENEFITS

Anecdotal evidence suggests EFT is effective in addressing post-traumatic stress disorder, depression, anxiety, and other psychiatric conditions. Due to the strong link between mind and body, EFT may also relieve some physical symptoms that may have resulted from emotional causes. These conditions include cancer, heart disease, hypertension, obesity, and diabetes.

Research has shown EFT significantly decreases anxiety in individuals with anxiety disorders (Clond, 2016). Another study showed that EFT was no more effective in alleviating symptoms of post-traumatic stress disorder than other conventional and complementary modalities (Sebastian & Nelms, 2017). Other studies have shown that EFT is more effective than conventional methods at mitigating psychosocial issues. This same study found EFT was more effective at improving sleep hygiene and lessening symptoms of depression than diaphragmatic breathing and motivational interviewing (Nelms & Castel, 2016). Another study has shown EFT is effective in decreasing symptoms of depression and anxiety in those with eating disorders. This study did not show any changes in physical symptoms related to the eating disorder (Stapleton et al., 2017).

CONTRAINDICATIONS, PRECAUTIONS, AND SIDE EFFECTS

Precautions include the risk of some past negative emotions resurfacing. This is brief but required in order to take part in EFT. However, the idea behind stating these negative memories or emotions is to use the process of EFT to lessen the associated discomfort. EFT is contraindicated for those with moderately or severely impaired long-term memory, as memory will be used to recall memories for EFT. There are no side effects associated with EFT.

CREDENTIALING

No license or certification is required to train patients on the use of EFT. For those who wish to pursue this certification, there are two levels that consist of 48 hours of educational content along with 30 hours of practical experience through live training. The only prerequisite for entering the EFT certification is a degree in mental health or a related field (Church, 2012).

EMOTIONAL FREEDOM TECHNIQUES AND OCCUPATIONAL THERAPY

EFT can be practiced on patients without any license. Knowing the basics of EFT is sufficient to begin incorporating these techniques as a preparatory method in occupational therapy treatment sessions. Specifically, EFT is a good technique to train patients on for use within their daily lives. This is a good recommendation for patients who are looking for ways to independently work on their past traumas and psychiatric symptoms. For the safety of the patient, the practice of EFT with an instructor is indicated for patients with a history of intense trauma to work through. Patients can add this sequence to their self-care routines to improve mood and overall functional performance.

A session of EFT involves an instructor verbally guiding an individual through the EFT sequence, so EFT can be completed independent of an instructor after one session. Another option is for an individual to learn EFT through home study for independent practice.

BASICS OF EMOTIONAL FREEDOM TECHNIQUES

1. What part of your body do you feel your emotional issue the strongest?

2. Assess your subjective units of distress (SUD) level on a scale of 1 to 10, similar to that of the visual analog pain scale.

3. Insert the name of your problem into the setup statement: "Even though I have (this problem), I deeply and completely accept myself."

4. Using the tips of four fingers, tap continuously on the karate chop point while repeating the setup statement three times. The karate chop point is on the ulnar side of each hand just above the wrist (see Figure 19-1).

5. While repeating the reminder phrase, which is a shortened version of the setup statement, use both fingers to tap seven times on the other seven points:

   - At the innermost tip of each eyebrow
   - At the outermost edge of each eye
   - Underneath each eye
   - Underneath the nose
   - Below the lip at the chin
   - Just below each side of the clavicle
   - Underneath each armpit

6. Test your results with a second SUD level.

Repeat the process until your SUD level gets closer to zero (Church, 2012).

CONSIDERATIONS FOR PRACTICE

Therapists should use EFT with patients in a private area where they feel comfortable discussing sensitive, traumatic, or distressing topics. Therapists should provide patients with tissues, notebooks, and writing utensils so they can record their thoughts, take notes on the EFT sequence, and form affirmations to help identify and work through difficult emotions. Therapists need to have some prior knowledge about their patient's personal history, which they can obtain during the first session. Therapists can then use this information to help patients understand the root of uncomfortable emotions and the internal response they may have had in response to certain events.

Therapists may write EFT-related goals in some of the following areas:

- Enhancing relaxation
- Practicing mindfulness
- Managing uncomfortable emotions
- Recognizing unhealthy behaviors and habits
- Developing plans to use healthy, productive routines and habits to cope with previously identified traumatic events
- Utilizing healthy tools to effectively manage responses to future traumatic or distressing events
- Understanding the mind-body connection and how it pertains to their life
- Incorporating EFT into a daily self-care routine

CHAPTER 20

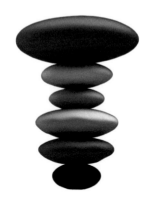

Eye Movement Desensitization and Reprocessing

Eye Movement Desensitization and Reprocessing (EMDR) is a form of psychotherapy used to help a person reprocess traumatic information until it no longer traumatizes them. EMDR is a noninvasive way to facilitate a person's ability to adapt when processing information. This reprocessing allows a person to gain insight into the reality of the traumatic situation, while also releasing themself from the shame, guilt, or blame surrounding the situation. This may involve someone having the realization the traumatic event is over, that they are currently safe, or that it will not happen again. This sense of safety allows the person to live in the present moment and take control of their life again.

EMDR uses an eight-phase approach to address a person's traumatic issues. These phases include history, preparation, assessment, desensitization, installation, body scan, closure, and re-evaluation.

Ferri, B. *Complementary Health Approaches*
for Occupational Therapists (pp. 97 100).
© 2021 Taylor & Francis Group.

In this instance, the terms processing and reprocessing do not refer to talking about the traumatic event. Rather, they involve analyzing negative self-talk the individual believes to be true and reframing the thoughts. This is immediately followed by self-reports of eye movements (also known as *taps* or *tones*). Once a person self-reports the presence (or absence) of these eye movements, the practitioner will provide sets of eye movements or other forms of stimulation to shift the person's focus. The effectiveness of these eye movements are evaluated before and after a session using a 1 to 10 scale of emotional distress, referred to as subjective units of distress (Eye Movement Desensitization and Reprocessing International Association, 2018).

BENEFITS

EMDR, due to its psychotherapy background, was initially developed to address the symptoms of post-traumatic stress disorder; however, its purpose has expanded during its time in practice. Research indicates EMDR is effective in improving trauma-associated symptoms related to comorbid psychiatric diagnoses, including psychosis, bipolar disorder, major depressive disorder, anxiety disorders, substance use disorders, and chronic pain disorders (Valiente-Gomez et al., 2017).

Another study detailed that EMDR caused a rapid decrease in symptoms of trauma. Participants in this same study reported a decrease in negative emotions, along with the vividness of persistently disturbing images (Shapiro, 2014). When tested on individuals with obsessive-compulsive disorder, EMDR proved to be no more effective at reducing symptoms of anxiety than cognitive behavioral therapy (Marsden et al., 2018).

Research showed EMDR yielded a clinically significant improvement in depressive symptoms. These findings were despite highly variable mood ratings throughout the course of the study (Wood et al., 2018). EMDR also showed a decreased amount of craving, fear, and depression, along with an improvement of emotion regulation and levels of self-esteem in those with substance use disorders (Pilz et al., 2017).

CONTRAINDICATIONS, PRECAUTIONS, AND SIDE EFFECTS

Precautions include risk of some discomfort when talking about past negative memories. Because EMDR must take place over several sessions (upwards of 8 to 10 sessions) before seeing results, this discomfort may be too much for some to tolerate. However, the discomfort is likely to be short-term if the individual completes the full, recommended course of EMDR as per their practitioner.

EMDR is contraindicated in patients with cognitive deficits and intellectual disabilities. This is because the modality relies on participation in self-reporting along with changing negative self-talk.

CREDENTIALING

Certification is required to practice EMDR. This certification is only available to individuals with an active certification and license in a mental health field. This must be accompanied by an educational training, along with 50 clinical EMDR sessions on patients. These requirements must be supplemented by 20 hours of EMDR consultation from an approved consultant who has completed their training and subsequent certification (Eye Movement Desensitization and Reprocessing International Association, 2018).

EYE MOVEMENT DESENSITIZATION AND REPROCESSING AND OCCUPATIONAL THERAPY

Individuals who possess the certification in EMDR and wish to incorporate it into occupational therapy treatment can do so. Due to the nature of the sessions, including traumatic disclosures along with the close attention needed to analyze eye movements, private practice is the best setting for this modality. Therapists who work in private practice with a psychiatric population would be best suited to use EMDR on patients.

This modality can be combined with lifestyle redesign, symptom management, emotion regulation, productive leisure, community engagement, along with a variety of other functional skills. This will assist the practitioner in maximizing gains for the patients on whom they perform EMDR.

CONSIDERATIONS FOR PRACTICE

Therapists trained in EMDR need to use inspected and well-maintained equipment, such as light bars, LED tactile pulsars, and more, to assist in implementing this modality. Therapists should use EMDR with patients in a private area where they feel comfortable discussing sensitive, traumatic, or distressing topics. Therapists should be sure to evaluate patients carefully before using EMDR. Therapists need to use this modality to target distressing emotions and later reshape them into positive (or neutral) beliefs that do not negatively impact their function. Therapists must properly store EMDR equipment to maintain the integrity of the devices. Therapists will need to remain up to date on best practices related to the use of each EMDR tool.

Therapists may write EMDR-related goals in some of the following areas:

- Managing uncomfortable emotions
- Recognizing unhealthy behaviors and habits
- Enhancing relaxation
- Practicing mindfulness
- Discovering traumatic events
- Developing plans to use healthy, productive routines and habits
- Understanding the mind-body connection and how it pertains to their life

CHAPTER 21

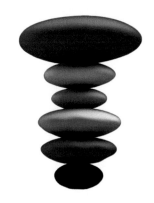

Guided Imagery

Guided imagery is a type of relaxation technique that can be used to calm both the body and the mind in order to decrease stress levels. Those who practice guided imagery use their ability to focus on pleasant sensations (e.g., images, feelings, smells, sounds, tastes) to lessen the intensity of negative memories or feelings. Guided imagery can be done by simply picturing things that make you happy (Figure 21-1). Guided imagery sessions can also be led by instructors or practiced through audio scripts. In the latter option, there are usually locations to choose from, such as beaches, forests, deserts, meadows, or waterfalls. If you are leading the practice yourself, you have the option to picture any place you find calming that may include childhood locations or places unique to your life (Cleveland Clinic, 2019).

Ferri, B. *Complementary Health Approaches*
for Occupational Therapists (pp. 101-105).
© 2021 Taylor & Francis Group.

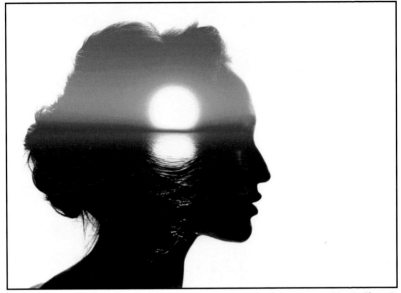

Figure 21-1. Guided imagery involves the visualization of calming scenes. Max4e Photo/ Shutterstock.com

BENEFITS

Anecdotal evidence suggests guided imagery can help increase self-control, sleep quality, immune system function, quality of life, and confidence. Additional anecdotal evidence states guided imagery can assist in decreasing depression, stress, anxiety, pain, nausea, blood pressure, and respiratory difficulties.

Research shows that guided imagery is effective in reducing nonmusculoskeletal pain (Posadzki et al., 2012). Another study showed the effectiveness of guided imagery in reducing food cravings and increasing physical activity while decreasing subjective reports of stress (Giacobbi et al., 2018). Research also demonstrated when individuals with fibromyalgia participated in guided imagery with hypnosis, they reported a decrease in pain, psychological distress, and disability status along with an improvement of health-related quality of life (Zech et al., 2017).

One study examined the impact of guided imagery on individuals 6 months after they had undergone total knee replacements. Results indicated participants experienced an increase in gait velocity and a decrease in pain scores after 3 weeks of guided imagery. Hair cortisol concentration was also significantly lower 6 months after surgery, indicating it played a role in lowering stress levels (Jacobson et al., 2016).

Contraindications, Precautions, and Side Effects

There have been some reports of guided imagery causing an increase in psychiatric symptoms in those individuals with a history of trauma. Side effects associated with an increase in psychiatric symptoms may include anxiety, intrusive thoughts, or disturbing images.

This modality is contraindicated for individuals who find that guided imagery brings about intrusive thoughts or disturbing memories that cannot be lessened. It is important to ask individuals with a trauma history about this and assess their willingness for participation, if these side effects have occurred. Guided imagery is also contraindicated for individuals who are actively psychotic or delirious, have dementia, lack expressive communication skills, or those who lack the ability to engage in abstract thought. These factors make it difficult for an individual to follow instructions or engage in images when prompted by another individual (Cleveland Clinic, 2019).

Credentialing

There are no licenses associated with guided imagery, nor are any licenses or certifications required to assist someone in performing guided imagery. There are certifications individuals can pursue if they are interested in receiving more training. The Academy for Guided Imagery and other online institutions offer such trainings that can be completed online or in-person, often on a self-paced basis.

Guided Imagery and Occupational Therapy

Interested practitioners can begin using guided imagery in their therapy practice at any time, as long as it is practiced on patients after assessing their risk for side effects. Some preparation will be needed, such as finding audio recordings or scripts for patient use. Guided imagery can be used in hospitals, nursing homes, outpatient facilities, and any other setting where therapy is provided. This can be used in a group format or individually with patients. Guided imagery can be incorporated into sessions as a preparatory activity to help improve performance in functional activities.

Practitioners can also structure the room to complement the relaxation process. This may include using ambient sounds, calming scents, smaller lights, and other small sensory modifications to deepen the practice of guided imagery further. This will help patients to feel more immersed in their environment, while simultaneously masking any distractions from the room.

BASICS OF GUIDED IMAGERY

Get into a relaxed position where you will be comfortable for some time. If you think lying down would put you to sleep, sit with your legs crossed or recline in a comfortable chair. Position yourself so you are comfortable and not distracted.

Use diaphragmatic breathing and close your eyes by breathing in peace and breathing out stress. Let your stomach expand and contract with your breath. If you find your shoulders rising and falling, you may be carrying tension in the body and not breathing in a fully relaxed way.

Once you are relaxed, imagine yourself in the midst of the most relaxing environment you can think of. For some people, this may be floating in the cool, clear waters off a tropical island with people bringing you drinks and nice music playing in the background. Some might like to picture themselves sitting by a fire in a secluded snowy cabin deep in the woods while sipping hot cocoa and reading the latest bestseller, wrapped in a blanket and wearing slippers. Some people may want to recall a time when they felt relaxed, a vividly described scene from a book they love, or the way they imagine places they have always wanted to visit.

As you imagine your scene, try to involve all of your senses. What does it look like? How does it feel? What special scents are involved? Do you hear the roar of a fire, the splash of a waterfall, or the sounds of chipper birds? Make your vision so real you can even taste it! (Noticing these details in your daily life is a way to increase your mindfulness and bring lasting stress management benefits as well.)

Stay here for as long as you like. Enjoy your "surroundings," and let yourself be far from what stresses you. When you're ready to come back to reality, count back from 10 or 20, and tell yourself that when you get to "one," you'll feel serene and alert, and enjoy the rest of your day. When you return, you'll feel calmer and refreshed, like returning from a mini-vacation, but you won't have left the room (Scott, 2018)!

CONSIDERATIONS FOR PRACTICE

Therapists should dedicate a private, quiet place where patients can participate in guided imagery. Therapists can modify the setting if there is limited space or availability by providing a comfortable temperature with essential oils, soothing music, blankets, along with comfortable chairs and mats. In order to provide comprehensive care, therapists must have some prior knowledge about their patient's history to ensure that they are providing trauma-specific care and remaining sensitive to certain triggers or past events. This means that therapists must complete an evaluation before beginning any form of guided imagery. In order to implement this modality, therapists need to prepare specific written scripts or video scripts to help guide patients through the process. Patients or therapists may opt for a beach, forest, park, or personally meaningful setting.

Therapists may write guided imagery–related goals in some of the following areas:

- Improving emotional awareness and management of uncomfortable emotions
- Enhancing relaxation
- Practicing mindfulness
- Improving body awareness
- Understanding the mind-body connection and how it pertains to their life
- Incorporating guided imagery into a daily self-care routine

CHAPTER 22

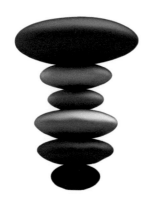

Herbalism

Herbalism is a modality implemented as part of Traditional Chinese Medicine (TCM). Herbal medicine uses raw and unpurified extracts of whole plants to address the underlying causes of disease. These extracts can be taken in a variety of forms but are popularly used in blends of several herbs (Figure 22-1). **Crude herbs** are dried, cut, and sifted, while **powders** are crude herbs that have been ground. **Capsules** are crude herbs placed in a tube to be swallowed like a pill. **Teas** are aqueous extracts taken from crude herbs or powders. **Tinctures** are herbs soaked in a drawing solution. Solutions can vary in strength, for example, one part alcohol and two parts herb (1:2) or one part alcohol and five parts herb (1:5). **Granules** are the solid residue formed after herbs are cooked (Tillotson, 2001).

The idea of combinations in conventional medicine, also called *polypharmacy*, is discouraged due to chemical interactions. This principle is what makes herbal medicine more versatile, but consumers must also be cautious. Diagnostic methods associated with TCM govern use of

Ferri, B. *Complementary Health Approaches*
for Occupational Therapists (pp. 107-111).
© 2021 Taylor & Francis Group.

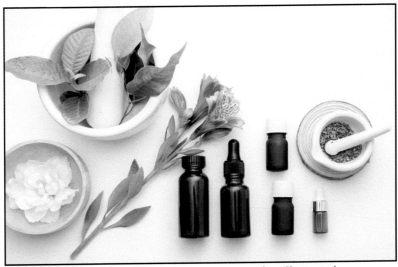

Figure 22-1. Herbal medicine uses whole plant extracts. paulynn/Shutterstock.com

specific herbs. These diagnostic principles include addressing the underlying cause and may lead herbalists to recommend several different herbs to address the whole picture of a patient's illness (Vickers et al., 2001).

BENEFITS

The benefits of herbal formulas vary largely depending on the herb and its classification. It is difficult to review specific research due to the high number of herbs on record.

Siberian ginseng root bark and jiaogulan leaves are examples of **adaptogenic herbs**, used to strengthen the body. **Alterative herbs** increase waste elimination through the liver, large intestine, lungs, lymph, skin, and kidneys. Some alterative herbs are burdock root, dandelion root, red clover blossom, and tu fu ling rhizome. **Amphoteric herbs** balance hyperactive or hypoactive organs and bodily processes. Some amphoteric herbs include licorice root, cordyceps mushroom, and Siberian ginseng.

Antimicrobial herbs, including isatis root, oregano, and horseradish, help to reduce bacterial and fungal activity within the body. **Antiseptic herbs**, including tea tree oil and oregano oil, prohibit external bacterial activity. **Aphrodisiac herbs**, such as potency bark and ashwagandha root, stimulate sexual drive. **Demulcent herbs** soothe and protect damaged internal tissues. A common demulcent herb is slippery elm bark. **Diuretic herbs** stimulate the removal of fluids from the body by increasing the flow of urine. Diuretic herbs include dandelion leaf and coffee bean.

Emollient herbs, such as olive oil, soften and soothe the skin. **Emmenagogue herbs** are herbs that stimulate and promote healthy menstruation. Emmenagogue herbs include turmeric root and chaste tree berry. **Expectorant herbs**, such as licorice root, assist in the expulsion of mucus from the lungs. **Hemostatic herbs** assist the body in stopping blood flow. Tien chi root is a hemostatic herb.

Stimulant laxative herbs increase activity of the lower bowel muscles. Rhubarb root is one stimulant laxative. **Bulk-forming laxative herbs**, such as flaxseed, increase the water content and size of stool. **Nervine herbs** calm and soothe the nervous system. Common nervine herbs are milky oat seed and skullcap.

Stimulant herbs increase overall mental and metabolic activity. Stimulant herbs include ephedra, coffee, and ginseng root. **Tonic herbs** serve to tone and strengthen the immune system, slow the aging process, and strengthen specific organs. Tonic herbs include Siberian ginseng and astragalus root (Tillotson, 2001).

The U.S. National Library of Medicine has compiled information on the uses of many common herbs. This information can be found at https://medlineplus.gov/druginfo/herb_All.html.

CONTRAINDICATIONS, PRECAUTIONS, AND SIDE EFFECTS

The risks associated with each herb vary largely and should be researched thoroughly before use on any patient, even those who are medically stable. Most risks associated with consumption of herbs are related to their interactions with prescription pharmaceuticals. This can cause a synergistic effect that can result in life-threatening injury or even death.

Below are just some interactions between chemical medications and herbs, but this is not an all-inclusive list. Echinacea can cause hepatotoxicity when taken with anabolic steroids, methotrexate, amiodarone, and ketoconazole. Feverfew can take on an inhibitory effect when taken with nonsteroidal, anti-inflammatory drugs. This will make both medications seemingly ineffective and may cause someone to increase the dosage on one or both, leading to life-threatening injuries. Individuals who take feverfew, garlic, ginseng, ginkgo biloba, or ginger with warfarin sodium may experience delays in blood clotting.

Taking ginseng with phenelzine sulfate can cause headaches, tremors, and manic episodes. Taking St. John's wort with antidepressants, such as monoamine oxidase inhibitors or serotonin reuptake inhibitors, can cause synergistic effects. These medications are intended to improve symptoms of depression; however, symptoms of depression can worsen if these supplements and medications are combined. St. John's wort can also decrease the effectiveness of antiretroviral medications, digoxin, theophylline, cyclosporine, and oral contraceptives.

Valerian and kava kava should not be taken with barbiturates due to the risk of excessive sedation and suppression of the central nervous system. Kyushin, licorice, plantain, uzara root, hawthorn, and ginseng should not be taken with digoxin due to their interference with potency in blood levels. Evening primrose oil and borage should not be taken with anticonvulsant medications, as this will lower the threshold for seizures. Echinacea and zinc should not be taken with corticosteroids and cyclosporine, as the herbs will lessen the effects of the chemical immunosuppressants.

Kelp should not be taken with thyroxine, as the iodine content in kelp may interfere with thyroid levels. Licorice should not be taken with spironolactone, as licorice can block the diuretic effect of the chemical medication. Karela and ginseng should not be taken by anyone with diabetes or anyone taking insulin, sulfonylureas, or biguanides, as these herbs can impact blood glucose levels.

Herbal medicine in any form is contraindicated for patients who are taking several prescription pharmaceuticals, as this can cause serious interactions (Vickers et al., 2001). The U.S. National Library of Medicine has compiled information regarding dosages and chemical interactions of many common herbs. This information can be found at https://medlineplus.gov/druginfo/herb_All.html.

CREDENTIALING

Herbal medicine can only be practiced with a license and certification. The American Herbalists Guild and American Association of Naturopathic Physicians both provide this education and certification. Certification through the American Herbalists Guild consists of 1,200 hours of education along with 400 hours of clinical internships (Tillotson, 2001). Licenses to practice TCM and naturopathic medicine also include herbal medicine in their scope of practice. Some acupuncture training programs include education on herbal medicine and the option to pursue a dual certification.

HERBALISM AND OCCUPATIONAL THERAPY

The use of herbal medicine should not be combined with occupational therapy practice unless a therapist has undergone extensive training in the practice of herbal medicine. Only after this training and subsequent certification and/or licensure has been attained can an occupational therapist use herbal medicine in their practice. Even then, therapists should be sure to educate their patients to consult their primary care physician to review all medications for potential interactions.

This modality is best practiced with patients individually to allow for adequate evaluation and consultation. Private practice or outpatient clinics are likely the best setting for this modality to be used. Herbal medicine routines can be an aspect of self-care training and symptom management that occupational therapists assist their patients with developing if they are interested. Herbal medicine can be combined with lifestyle redesign, symptom management, emotion regulation, productive leisure, community engagement, along with a variety of other functional skills.

CONSIDERATIONS FOR PRACTICE

Therapists trained in herbalism are able to provide patients with herbal recommendations based on the symptoms they present with. It would be beneficial for therapists to have herbs at their clinic location to ensure that patients are getting quality herbs from a safe retailer. This modality mainly consists of counseling patients regarding their current health habits, so therapists may want to offer their patients a semiprivate location where they can discuss symptoms, lifestyle choices, and traumatic events that may be sensitive.

Therapists may write herbalism-related goals in some of the following areas:

- Enhancing relaxation
- Managing uncomfortable emotions
- Reducing inflammation
- Increasing functional performance
- Improving sleep hygiene
- Complying with herbal recommendations per therapist direction
- Using good safety and judgment by following recommendations per manufacturer and consulting doctor regarding potential medication interactions
- Recording symptoms after taking to report to therapist
- Understanding the benefits and risks associated with herbal supplements
- Using herbs in accordance with a self-care routine

CHAPTER 23

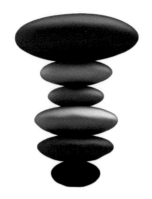

Hypnotherapy

Hypnotherapy, also known as *hypnosis*, is a modality where a practitioner assists an individual in entering a state of heightened focus and concentration. This state of focus is used to access the unconscious mind so that the practitioner can then work on one specific issue the individual may be experiencing (Figure 23-1). This process consists of mental imagery and verbal repetition to increase the individual's suggestibility. By making an individual more suggestible, the hope is to achieve a deeper sense of mental and bodily relaxation.

A common myth about hypnosis is that the hypnotized individual loses control and is no longer able to end the session if they desire. The opposite is true—the individual is actually able to talk, move, and behave as they normally would. The only difference is a more relaxed state than the individual would experience at baseline. Hypnosis typically requires several sessions to achieve the desired effect, making this method a good option for those who expect immediate results (American Society of Clinical Hypnotists [ASCH], 2019).

Ferri, B. *Complementary Health Approaches for Occupational Therapists* (pp. 113-117).
© 2021 Taylor & Francis Group.

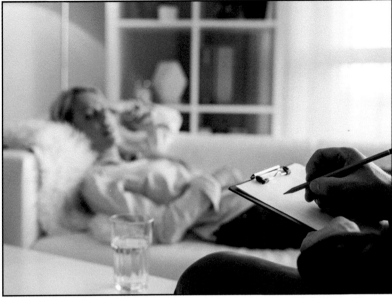

Figure 23-1. Unlike the well-known myth, individuals remain in control during hypnotherapy. Kaspars Grinvalds/Shutterstock.com

BENEFITS

Anecdotal evidence suggests hypnotherapy can be effective for managing pain, phobias, hot flashes, chemotherapy side effects, weight control, speech disorders, sexual problems, alcoholism, psychiatric symptoms, and difficult behaviors (ASCH, 2019).

There is not much research on the use of hypnosis; however, existing research has demonstrated positive results. One research study showed that, when compared to nicotine replacement therapy, hypnosis was significantly more effective at creating nonsmokers after 12 weeks of sessions (Hasan et al., 2014). Another study demonstrated the effectiveness of hypnosis in increasing self-esteem and optimism while decreasing anxiety and distress after 12 sessions. After 24 sessions, increased self-esteem and optimism were still reported (Tellez et al., 2017). Another research study showed hypnosis significantly reduced bowel inflammation and enhanced health-related quality of life in individuals with inflammatory bowel disease (Szigethy, 2015).

CONTRAINDICATIONS, PRECAUTIONS, AND SIDE EFFECTS

Hypnotherapy is contraindicated for those individuals with severe mental illness, as the process and perceived loss of control could cause an increase in psychiatric symptoms.

An individual who undergoes hypnosis rarely experiences side effects. Precautions associated with hypnosis include an increased risk for temporary headache, sedation, dizziness, anxiety, or the creation of false memories that can occur after a session (ASCH, 2019).

CREDENTIALING

Hypnotherapy can only be practiced after receiving the appropriate training and obtaining a license. Hypnotherapy training is only available to those individuals who possess a master's degree and a license to practice clinical psychology, medicine, social work, or marriage and family therapy. ASCH believes these professions provide adequate foundations in mental health and psychology to succeed in meeting the competencies of hypnotherapy (2019). Training in hypnotherapy consists of 40 hours of educational classes followed by 20 hours of consulting with and practicing hypnosis on a currently certified hypnotist. A practitioner must document 2 years practicing hypnosis on patients before they can obtain certification.

HYPNOTHERAPY AND OCCUPATIONAL THERAPY

Occupational therapists can only practice hypnotherapy if they have another degree in one of the required fields along with the appropriate certification and licensure. A private practice or outpatient setting where there is ample space and an increased likelihood of a quiet, distraction-free environment would be best for the practice of hypnotherapy. Therapists should first evaluate patients to determine hypnotherapy is safe to perform.

Hypnotherapy can be completed as a main modality in sessions or a preparatory activity to encourage relaxation for engagement in functional tasks later. This modality can be combined with lifestyle redesign, life skills training, symptom management, emotion regulation, vocational training, and more.

BASICS OF HYPNOTHERAPY

Goal accomplishment script: You are a self-confident winner who accomplishes your goals. Your life is a series of successes. All of your experiences are potential opportunities. You can accomplish anything. Your only limitation is your imagination and you now let your imagination go free. You are very clear about what you want out of life and you get what you want out of life. You have the self-discipline to stick with your goals until they are accomplished. You allow only positive and winning thoughts to flow through your mind. You are filled with optimism and enthusiasm in pursuing your goals to fruition. You are a goal-oriented winner. You accomplish all of your goals. You feel an intense inner drive to reach your goals, to accomplish, and to win.

Healing script: You are surrounded by a divine blue healing light that is flowing through all of your cells, healing you quickly and completely. You have the power and ability to accelerate the healing of your body. Your body is filled with positive healing energy and your healing is now accelerated. Each breath of air you take into your body contains the divine healing prana. Your mind is all powerful and you now use it to heal yourself of all imperfections that are now in your body (such as . . .). You are now healed and your body has returned to a perfect state. From this moment forward, you choose only perfect health—mentally, physically, and spiritually. Perfect health is your divine right and you now manifest perfect health. Each moment, each second, each hour, you move rapidly toward total healing of yourself. You are healed. You now focus upon the healing power of the universe—mentally, physically, and spiritually.

Prosperity script: Begin programming your computer now. Negative thoughts or negative suggestions have no influence over you at any level of your mind. You reject all thoughts and suggestions detrimental to your health, wealth, and happiness. The inner kingdom of your mind is universal. Your thoughts are success power reactors. Your brain waves are tuned to natural success frequencies. You are highly receptive to conditions and circumstances beneficial to your health, wealth, and happiness. It is your natural right to be rich. You accept this right at all times. You program your master computer daily to alert your conscious mind to any financial opportunities that will enhance your personal gain. Programming is effective now. This input is a powerful money reaction circuit. It functions to attract money in your daily life.

(continued)

BASICS OF HYPNOTHERAPY (CONTINUED)

It also acts as a money multiplier. When you use your money freely in exchange for values, it returns to you multiplied many times. Money attraction is a constant function of your computer. It constantly flows in your life. Money will never be harmful to you. It will always return to you in a good way. You will always have a healthy, positive attitude about money. Money is never a problem to you because you concentrate on the solution. You negotiate with money in a highly profitable way each day in every way possible. Your business is growing each day. Your sales are increasing in every way. Money is constantly flowing and circulating in your life (ASCH, 2019).

CONSIDERATIONS FOR PRACTICE

Therapists should use hypnotherapy with patients in a private area where they feel comfortable discussing sensitive, traumatic, or distressing topics. Therapists should offer support for patients as they help identify and work through difficult emotions or past traumas. Therapists need to have some prior knowledge about their patient's personal history, which they can obtain during the first session, in order to best inform practice. Therapists do not need additional tools or resources for this modality, aside from having a standard hypnotherapy script prepared.

Therapists may write hypnotherapy-related goals in some of the following areas:

- Developing plans to use healthy, productive routines and habits to cope with any trauma
- Managing uncomfortable emotions
- Recognizing unhealthy behaviors and habits
- Enhancing relaxation
- Practicing mindfulness
- Utilizing healthy tools to effectively manage responses to future traumatic or distressing events
- Understanding the mind-body connection and how it pertains to their life
- Incorporating the principles of hypnotherapy into a daily self-care routine

Chapter 24

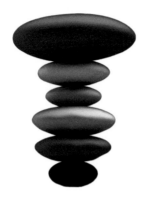

Iridology

Iridology is a modality that uses analysis of the iris to reveal the location of inflammation, poor elimination, and over-acidity within the body. This analysis can also tell the body's constitution, inherent weaknesses, levels of health, and the changes that the body will go through according to an individual's lifestyle (Figure 24-1). Iridology is a noninvasive mechanism that sheds light into areas of health where a practitioner can coach an individual to improve.

Iridology is not a method of diagnosis nor is it a method of treatment, though iridology practitioners do have training in holistic recommendations. Iridology practitioners will typically provide diet recommendations, lifestyle changes, and vitamin, mineral, or herbal supplements to assist the individual in mitigating risk factors and issues as determined by the iris analysis. Until several decades ago, iridology was incorporated into the training of allopathic medical doctors. Due to their scope of practice, they were able to use findings from iridology to assist in diagnosis and treatment of their patients (Petersen, 2017).

Ferri, B. *Complementary Health Approaches for Occupational Therapists* (pp. 119-123). © 2021 Taylor & Francis Group.

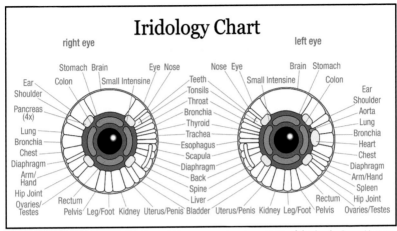

Figure 24-1. Parts of the iris are thought to represent various parts of the body. Peter Hermes Furian/Shutterstock.com

BENEFITS

Little research is present regarding the effectiveness of iridology. Research that does exist has mixed outcomes, as iridology is neither widely used nor well understood. Studies have tested the ability of iridology practitioners to predict signs pointing toward already made, official diagnoses.

In 110 subjects, an iridology practitioner correctly identified three cases of cancer out of 68 subjects who had cancer (Munstedt et al., 2005). Another research study showed an iridology practitioner was able to correctly identify 70% of subjects with hearing loss (Stearn & Swanepoel, 2006).

CONTRAINDICATIONS, PRECAUTIONS, AND SIDE EFFECTS

There are no risks, contraindications, or precautions associated with iridology. This noninvasive modality consists of iris analysis and offers no intervention or diagnostic process.

CREDENTIALING

Individuals interested in using iridology on patients do not need a health care background. There is no licensure to practice iridology, but a certification is required. The International Iridology Practitioners Association states certification consists of completing a training program, basic anatomy courses, 10 iris analyses, and an examination (International Iridology Practitioners Association, n.d.).

BASICS OF IRIDOLOGY

Lacunae: Oval-shaped areas with fewer colored fibers, or fibers lacking color altogether. There are many types of lacunae, but the presence of any lacunae typically indicates deficits in the lymphatic system and/or endocrine system and over-acidity accumulated in the body.

Tetanic rings: Circular arcs toward the middle of the iris. The presence of tetanic rings typically indicates a predisposition to spasms and contractions, placing an individual at risk for heart diseases, anxiety, and insomnia.

Radii solaris: A large ring-like shape with rays coming from the center of the iris. The presence of radii solaris typically indicates a predisposition to cognitive deficits, including memory, attention, and potential "mental breakdown."

Lymphatic constitution: A blue iris with loose and wavy fibers. Individuals with this lymphatic constitution typically have issues associated with the lymphatic system, including tonsil irritations, spleen and appendix deficits, swollen lymph nodes, eczema, acne, dry and flaky skin, dandruff, asthma, bronchitis, sinusitis, diarrhea, arthritis, mucous discharge, eye irritations, and fluid retention.

Hematogenic constitution: A brown or deep brown iris with no other colors or major fiber changes visible; small differentiations in iris fibers are present upon closer examination with lighter areas or areas with sparse fibers indicating inflammation. These individuals have a tendency toward developing radii solaris. Individuals with this constitution typically have issues, such as anemia, mineral deficiencies, blood diseases, muscle spasms, arthritis, endocrine disorders, swollen glands, constipation, colonic tumors, dyspepsia, dairy intolerance, ulcers, diabetes, circulatory disorders, and malfunctions of liver, gallbladder, and pancreas.

Biliary constitution: A blue background with a brown overlay, making for a hazel or greenish iris. This can be often confused with the hematogenic constitution due to the lack of major fiber changes. Individuals with this constitution typically have issues with constipation, flatulence, colitis, hypoglycemia, diabetes, blood diseases, gallstones, gastrointestinal weakness, and disorders of the liver, gallbladder, pancreas, and bile duct (Petersen, 2017) (Figure 24-2).

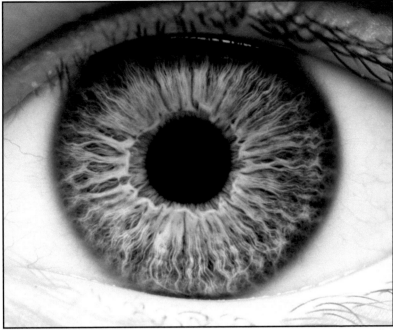

Figure 24-2. Iridology uses an iris analysis to determine bodily weaknesses. Bradley Blackburn/Shutterstock.com

IRIDOLOGY AND OCCUPATIONAL THERAPY

Iridology can only be completed by those who possess a certification as an iridologist. A private practice or outpatient setting where there is ample space and an increased likelihood of a quiet, distraction-free environment would be best for iridology. This can be combined with lifestyle redesign, symptom management, and more as a method to improve the health and wellness of an individual.

CONSIDERATIONS FOR PRACTICE

Therapists trained in iridology need special magnifying devices with bright lights to allow them to analyze their patients' eyes. Therapists should use iridology with patients in a private area where they feel comfortable with this physical examination. Therapists need to educate their patients that this modality cannot diagnose or treat any medical conditions, rather this modality can potentially help individuals lower the levels of inflammation in their bodies and build healthy lifestyles to prevent illness.

Therapists will need notebooks and pens in order to write out plans and health recommendations for their patients. Therapists must properly store iridology equipment to maintain the integrity of the devices.

Therapists may write iridology-related goals in some of the following areas:

- Recognizing unhealthy behaviors and habits
- Modifying diet in a way that supports a healthy lifestyle
- Creating an exercise plan to increase physical activity and lower bodily inflammation
- Using health recommendations daily as part of a self-care routine
- Developing plans to increase compliance with healthy, productive routines and habits
- Understanding the mind-body connection and how it pertains to their life

CHAPTER 25

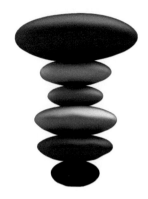

Light Therapy

Light therapy is a modality that uses LED light units to provide red, blue, and infrared lights to all layers of the skin along with the muscles and bones (Figure 25-1). The wavelengths used in light therapy are intended to stimulate circulation and decrease pain by stimulating the photoreceptors of the skin to increase energy production.

Near infrared light is 750 to 1400 nm. This range is ideal for reaching the level of the bone and for addressing issues associated with internal organs, glands, bone, cartilage, ligaments, and deep muscle tissue. Visible red light is 630 to 700 nm and can reach tissue 10 mm below the surface. This is good for addressing issues associated with the muscle, fascia, and skin. Visible blue light is 430 to 500 nm and can penetrate tissue 5 mm below the surface. This is ideal for addressing issues associated with the skin, including wounds, cuts, scars, abrasions, inflammation, infections, and skin abnormalities, such as eczema, acne, and psoriasis (Zarabi-Smith, 2013) (Figure 25-2).

Ferri, B. *Complementary Health Approaches for Occupational Therapists* (pp. 125-128). © 2021 Taylor & Francis Group.

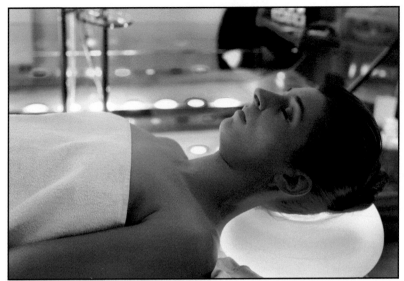

Figure 25-1. Different colored lights are intended to have various effects on the body and mind. Kzenon/Shutterstock.com

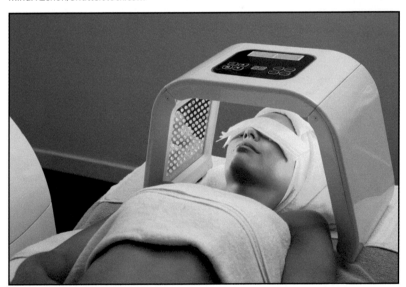

Figure 25-2. Visible blue light can address a range of skin issues. Dragon Images/Shutterstock.com

BENEFITS

Anecdotal evidence suggests light therapy can relieve minor pain, stiffness, and muscle spasms, while causing a temporary increase in local blood circulation. The majority of the research on physical deficits has been done on red and blue light. Other colors of the visible spectrum are available for use; however, there is limited evidence regarding their purpose for certain populations (Zarabi-Smith, 2013).

Research has shown that blue and red light are effective in regulating the autonomic nervous system, along with alleviating respiratory symptoms, tonsillitis, and displaced vertebrae (Elkina et al., 2013). Additional studies have been done proving the effectiveness of red and green light toward improving cognitive deficits in older adults (Paragas et al., 2019).

CONTRAINDICATIONS, PRECAUTIONS, AND SIDE EFFECTS

The use of soft lasers are approved and classified by the U.S. Food and Drug Administration, who have cleared soft lasers and the use of infrared energy as safe for use by qualified professionals. There are no side effects associated with the use of light therapy. Light therapy is contraindicated for individuals with circulatory issues or disorders. Individuals who receive light therapy on their face should have an eye mask, towel, or other barrier to shield their eyes, as the light can be damaging.

CREDENTIALING

No license is required to practice light therapy; however, a certification is required. Training for certification can be completed by those without licensure in a health care discipline. The first step toward certification is completion of anatomy and physiology followed by a satisfactory score on an anatomy exam. The full training consists of 60 self-study hours of educational content and an exam. This then qualifies an individual to receive certification through the Board of Advanced Natural Health Sciences and hold the credentials "CLET" or "CLT" after their name (Zarabi-Smith, 2013).

LIGHT THERAPY AND OCCUPATIONAL THERAPY

Only certified light therapists should practice light therapy. Light therapy would best be completed in a private practice or outpatient setting where there is ample space and an increased likelihood of a quiet, distraction-free environment. This modality is best completed individually. If this modality were to be used in a group setting, it would still be important to evaluate each patient to ensure their appropriateness for light therapy.

Light therapy can be completed as a main modality in sessions or as a preparatory activity to encourage improved blood flow, range of motion, and decreased pain levels for engagement in functional tasks later. Certain patients may be appropriate for training and education on home units, if they find success with this modality. It is important to ensure the reliability and source of home equipment is satisfactory for its intended purpose.

CONSIDERATIONS FOR PRACTICE

Therapists trained in light therapy need to use inspected and well-maintained equipment, such as LED light bars, light pads, wearable light apparatuses, and more, to assist in implementing this modality. Therapists should use light therapy with patients in a private area where they feel comfortable sitting for 30 to 90 minutes while receiving the lights. Due to the extended time that patients are sitting, they should have additional amenities, such as soothing music, calming aromas, comfortable blankets, pens and paper to track symptoms, or movies to watch. Therapists should be sure to evaluate patients carefully before using light therapy, since this modality is only applicable for certain symptoms and diagnoses. Therapists must also monitor patients closely (especially patients with poor sensation) to ensure that lights are not too hot, as this may cause burns. Therapists must properly store light therapy equipment to maintain the integrity of the devices. Aside from specific training in use of each tool, therapists should not need any other special preparation to use light therapy on patients.

Therapists may write light therapy–related goals in some of the following areas:

- Enhancing relaxation
- Tracking symptoms before and after light therapy sessions
- Improving range of motion
- Increasing endurance
- Reducing edema and general inflammation
- Decreasing pain levels
- Improving skin integrity and wound healing
- Increasing independence in transfers and functional mobility
- Understanding the risks and benefits of light therapy
- Managing difficult behaviors
- Developing plans to use healthy, productive routines and habits
- Comprehending the mind-body connection and how it pertains to their life

CHAPTER 26

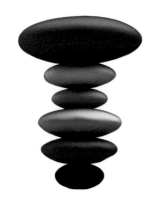

Massage Therapy

Massage therapy is a manual modality used to press, rub, and/or manipulate various parts of the body (Figure 26-1). There are different types of massage and each vary in the amount of pressure applied. Depending on the therapist, the massage may include oils, lotions, or other emollients to assist in manipulating muscles along with providing optimal relaxation.

Swedish massage is a gentle rubbing with circular motions and vibrations intended to both energize and relax. **Deep tissue massage** is a higher-pressure technique intended to target deep muscle and connective tissue. Deep tissue massage can be helpful for a range of overuse injuries along with chronic aches and pains. **Sports massage** is a lighter-pressure massage used to prevent or address injuries in athletes. **Trigger point massage** is a medium-pressure technique used to relieve tension in tight muscle fibers after long-standing overuse issues or injuries.

Ferri, B. *Complementary Health Approaches for Occupational Therapists* (pp. 129-132).
© 2021 Taylor & Francis Group.

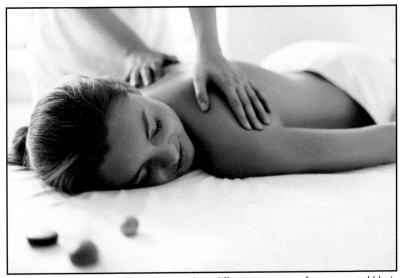

Figure 26-1. Each form of massage involves different amounts of pressure. puhhha/ Shutterstock.com

BENEFITS

Anecdotal evidence suggests massage therapy can assist in decreasing symptoms associated with anxiety disorders, preterm infancy, digestive disorders, arthritis, asthma, multiple sclerosis, Parkinson's disease, dementia, fibromyalgia, migraines, insomnia, myofascial pain syndrome, soft tissue injuries, skin conditions, and temporomandibular joint pain (Field, 2016).

Research suggests there is some evidence of massage's effectiveness in reducing pain of individuals with arthritis (Nelson & Churilla, 2017). Another study on surgical patients showed the effectiveness of massage in decreasing both generalized pain levels and pain local to the incision site (Kukimoto et al., 2017). When completed on preterm infants, massage benefits included increased vagal activity, increased gastric activity, improved neurodevelopment, and increased insulin levels. Additional benefits include a decreased risk of neonatal sepsis, lower neonatal stress, and a shorter hospital stay (Alvarez et al., 2017). Another research study indicated massage significantly reduced generalized pain or pain related to chemotherapy in individuals with cancer (Lee et al., 2015).

Massage also appears to be effective for general musculoskeletal pain or discomfort, unassociated with any diagnosis. A research study showed massage was effective for short-term pain reduction in those with acute lower back pain. The same study showed massage was effective in reducing pain and improving the function of those individuals with sub-acute and chronic lower back pain (Furlan et al., 2015).

CONTRAINDICATIONS, PRECAUTIONS, AND SIDE EFFECTS

Side effects depend on the type of massage received. Generalized soreness is common after a deep tissue massage, especially in relation to chronic injuries or massaged areas. Any significant discomfort felt during a massage should be mentioned to the therapist so they can modify their focus or the pressure they are providing. Precautions associated with massage therapy include an increased risk for clotting in individuals with a history of stroke or blood clotting. It is important for patients to mention this to their massage therapist before receiving a massage.

Massage is contraindicated for individuals with bleeding disorders, burns, open wounds, deep vein thrombosis, fractures, severe osteoporosis, severe thrombocytopenia, or who are taking blood-thinning medication (National Center for Complementary and Integrative Health, 2016c).

CREDENTIALING

In order to practice massage therapy, a license and certification as a massage therapist are required. This includes completing training for massage therapy, often involving a minimum of 500 hours educational content, along with a varying amount of clinically supervised practice hours.

Massage therapists can then pursue specialty certifications in sports massage, military veteran massage, clinical rehabilitative massage, massage for integrative health care, spa management, pain and palliative care, oncology massage, or reflexology. Chapter 33 will cover reflexology . Massage therapists also have the option to obtain their board certification through the National Certification Board for Therapeutic Massage and Bodywork (American Massage Therapy Association, 2019).

MASSAGE THERAPY AND OCCUPATIONAL THERAPY

Only those who possess a licensure and certification can provide massage therapy. Massage and manual techniques are within an occupational therapist's scope of practice and can be used as preparatory methods to decrease inflammation, pain, sensitivity, and stiffness, while increasing range of motion and flexibility. The effects of massage therapy can be utilized to improve engagement in therapeutic activities, therapeutic exercise, and/or functional tasks. Massage therapy is best suited for individual sessions on those who have first been evaluated.

In a psychiatric setting, self-massage methods may be used to encourage relaxation and assist with stress management. This can be done with small massagers bought from novelty stores, therapy putty, or other tools provided by a therapist.

Extensive massage therapy sessions would best be completed in a private practice or outpatient setting where there is ample space and privacy. However, massage on the upper extremity can be done with clothing on in hospitals, nursing homes, and home health.

CONSIDERATIONS FOR PRACTICE

Therapists trained in massage therapy should have a private area where patients can comfortably remove articles of clothing, as needed according to the body part(s) that are targeted. Some therapists may use tools (also called *instrument-assisted manual soft tissue massage*) to assist them in manipulating certain parts of a patient's body, such as muscles in the leg or back. Therapists should always determine a patient's current levels of pain, stiffness, and other symptomology before massaging. Therapists must provide individuals with continual instruction to ensure that patients maintain appropriate body positions and muscle relaxation throughout the process. Patients should also be able to verbalize pain or discomfort throughout the process, if this does occur. Most therapists will develop a specific plan regarding what body part to massage during each session but can alter the plan if patients present with varied symptoms before their session.

Therapists may write massage therapy–related goals in some of the following areas:

- Increasing endurance
- Enhancing strength and activity tolerance
- Improving postural symmetry and quality of movement
- Tracking symptoms before and after massage therapy
- Lowering pain levels
- Reducing inflammation
- Increasing range of motion to the neck, shoulder, hands, arms, legs, and torso (depending on area that receives massage therapy)
- Improving mobility and functional performance
- Using ergonomic posture and techniques along with joint protection strategies to maintain proper body alignment
- Increasing independence in transfers and functional mobility

CHAPTER 27

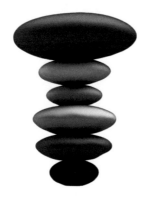

Meditation

Meditation is an umbrella term used to describe several ways of entering a relaxed state. This modality involves focusing attention on clearing the mind of external stimulus. This is intended to give a sense of calm, peace, and balance to improve both emotional and physical well-being (Figure 27-1). Types of meditation include guided imagery (see Chapter 21 for more information), mantra meditation, mindfulness meditation, and transcendental meditation. Meditation is also central to the practices of qigong (see Chapter 32 for more information), tai chi (see Chapter 35 for more information), and yoga (see Chapter 36 for more information).

Mantra meditation involves repeating a positive and inspiring word or phrase to assist with distraction and positive thinking. In **mindfulness meditation**, the focus is placed on awareness, living in the present, and on the flow of breath. As it may be difficult to distract from your thoughts, you may recognize what comes to mind and let it pass without giving it any more attention. **Transcendental meditation** involves repeating a mantra while allowing your body to enter a state of profound

Ferri, B. *Complementary Health Approaches for Occupational Therapists* (pp. 133-137).
© 2021 Taylor & Francis Group.

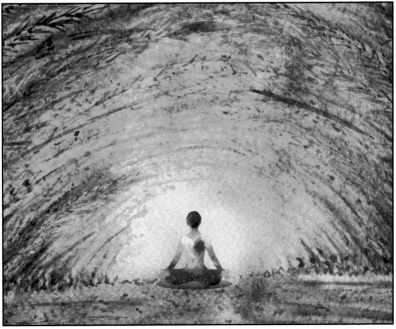

Figure 27-1. Guided imagery is a type of meditation. Benjavisa Ruangvaree Art/ Shutterstock.com

rest in order to achieve inner peace. By practicing transcendental meditation extensively, individuals can achieve this state with minimal effort or concentration (Mayo Clinic, 2017).

BENEFITS

Anecdotal evidence suggests meditation can benefit individuals with anxiety, asthma, cancer, chronic pain, depression, heart disease, high blood pressure, irritable bowel syndrome, sleep problems, nicotine addiction, ulcerative colitis, and migraines.

One research study showed that meditation was more effective than exercise at reducing chronic neck pain, generalized pain, and anxiety, while increasing feelings of altruism and life changes (Edwards & Loprinzi, 2018). Another research study found meditation was only slightly effective in decreasing chronic pain but significantly effective in reducing depressive symptoms and enhancing quality of life (Hilton et al., 2017). A different research study showed meditation improved pain tolerance and reduced medication usage in individuals with migraines. This same study showed meditation had no effect on pain sensitivity nor did it impact headache frequency (Wachholtz et al., 2017).

BASICS OF MEDITATION

Deep breathing: Focus all your attention on breathing, including the feeling and the sound as you inhale and exhale. When your attention wanders, gently remind yourself to focus on your breathing.

Body scanning: Focus attention on different parts of the body, including sensations, such as pain, tension, warmth, flexibility, or relaxation. When combined with deep breathing, you can imagine breathing heat into your body and turning the heat into relaxation that travels to whatever body part that needs it.

Mantras: Focus on repeating a mantra. You can create your own positive thought or use a religious one. This may include the Jesus prayer, the holy name of God prayer, the Om mantra, or others associated with certain religions.

Walking: Combining meditation with walking can boost the physical benefits associated with meditation. This can be used when you are walking in the forest, on a beach, or in a busy city. Slow down your walking pace and focus on each individual movement of your legs and feet. The destination is not important, rather the action words associated with each movement. For example, "lifting," "moving," and "placing" as they occur in real time.

Prayer: Spoken and written prayers associated with religion or created by yourself are good complements to meditation. Many resources are available if you would like to incorporate prayer into your meditation but are unsure how to.

Reading: Reading poetry, religious texts, or inspirational books can also be a part of your meditation. Giving yourself time to reflect on the meaning of what you are reading is important. This may include listening to relaxing music or music related to the texts you are reading. You may incorporate journaling about your reflections into this portion, if it feels natural.

Focus your love and gratitude: Focus all your attention on a sacred image or something that inspires you. Then, fill your thoughts with love, compassion, and gratitude. This may include closing your eyes to fully focus on the image.

Tips to remember: Meditation takes practice, as it is not intuitive for everyone. Experimenting with different types of meditation will help you find something you like and something that may be easier to engage in. Adapt your meditation practice to your present needs. There is no right or wrong way to meditate, all that exists is the way that feels most comfortable to you (Mayo Clinic, 2019).

Contraindications, Precautions, and Side Effects

Meditation that involves no movement is safe for everyone. Types of meditation that involve movement, such as tai chi, qigong, and yoga, should be used with caution or in modified forms for patients with physical impairments, especially significantly impaired balance, osteoporosis, or fractured bones. Side effects of meditation may include boredom, anxiety, depression, confusion, and disorientation in those individuals who are either not connected to the process or are not interested. Meditation is not contraindicated in any populations.

Credentialing

No licenses or certifications are required to practice meditation with patients. Those individuals interested in pursuing training and certification associated with meditation can find a variety of courses either online or in person.

Meditation and Occupational Therapy

Any occupational therapy practice can incorporate meditation. Settings where there is ample space and an increased likelihood of a quiet, distraction-free environment are best for meditation.

Occupational therapists may incorporate the use of meditation into occupational therapy treatment as a preparatory activity to encourage relaxation for engagement in functional tasks. This modality can be combined with lifestyle redesign, symptom management, emotion regulation, self-care training, leisure exploration, play, and more. Meditation can be performed either during individual sessions or group therapy, depending on patient needs, preferences, and ability to maintain a relatively quiet environment for the duration of the meditation.

Considerations for Practice

Therapists should dedicate a private, quiet place where patients can practice meditating. Therapists can modify the setting if there is limited space or availability by providing a comfortable temperature with essential oils, soothing music, blankets, along with comfortable chairs and mats. Therapists must have some prior knowledge about their patient's history to ensure that they are providing trauma-specific care and remaining sensitive to certain triggers or past events. This means that therapists must complete an evaluation before beginning any form of meditation. In order to implement this modality, therapists may need the help of specific written scripts or video scripts to help guide patients through the process, but more experienced therapists may be able to naturally lead patients through meditation.

Therapists may write meditation-related goals in some of the following areas:

- Practicing mindfulness
- Improving body awareness
- Understanding the mind-body connection and how it pertains to their life
- Increasing emotional awareness and management of uncomfortable emotions
- Enhancing relaxation
- Incorporating meditation into a daily self-care routine
- Regulating difficult behaviors

CHAPTER 28

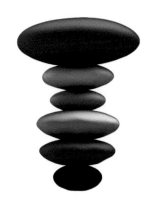

Music Therapy

Music therapy is a discipline that uses music to address the physical, emotional, cognitive, and social needs of patients through the therapeutic relationship. Music therapy consists of an evaluation process, followed by creating, singing to, moving to, or listening to music as a part of therapy (Figure 28-1). The main intention is to strengthen a patient's abilities in preparation for transferring these gains to functional areas.

Goals can include a patient's expression of emotion, improvement of mood, enhanced quality of life, improved communication, and more. Improved expressive communication is one of the most prevalent goals and effects of music therapy, as music can assist with reaching parts of the brain believed to be inactive (American Music Therapy Association, 2019).

Ferri, B. *Complementary Health Approaches*
for Occupational Therapists (pp. 139-142).
© 2021 Taylor & Francis Group.

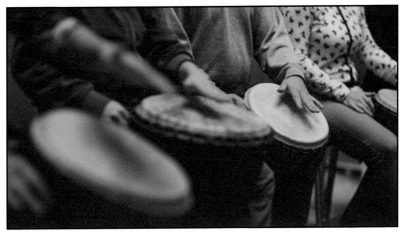

Figure 28-1. Music can be incorporated into many parts of treatment. l i g h t p o e t/ Shutterstock.com

BENEFITS

Anecdotal evidence suggests music therapy is most beneficial for individuals with depression, generalized stress and anxiety, autism spectrum disorder, and cancer.

Research has shown individuals receiving music therapy are more likely to see a decrease in depressive symptoms than those who do not receive therapy (Maratos et al., 2008). Another research study showed that music therapy significantly reduced stress, anxiety, and depression in healthy pregnant women (Chang et al., 2008).

One research study on individuals with mild Alzheimer's disease showed music therapy created significant improvements in memory, orientation, anxiety, and depression. This same study showed music therapy decreased the frequency and intensity of delirium, hallucinations, agitation, irritability, and verbal expression in those with moderate Alzheimer's disease (Gomez-Gallego & Gomez-Garcia, 2017).

Aside from its cognitive and emotional benefits, music therapy also has proven physical effects on the body. One research study showed that simple exposure to music caused a decrease in scores on the Morse fall scale, an outcome measure used to predict an individual's likelihood to fall (Chabot et al., 2019).

Contraindications, Precautions, and Side Effects

Precautions related to music therapy include the increased risk of repressed emotions or memories resurfacing. This may especially be harmful in a population with psychiatric or cognitive disorders. Music therapy may also cross the line into spirituality, causing potential conflict with the beliefs and practices of certain patients. Spiritual music is contraindicated for patients who have adverse reactions to or experiences with anything associated with spirituality.

In patients with cognitive deficits, music therapy may also instill false memories or confusion. This may result from the brain creating a memory associated with the melody they hear. Music therapy may also cause increased anxiety for individuals who do not like music or are not able to express their preference for certain music.

Credentialing

Those interested in practicing music therapy are required to complete an undergraduate degree program in music therapy to meet the minimum educational requirement for their field. There are three fieldwork opportunities associated with this degree path. Individuals may also opt for a master's degree program in the same field to further their knowledge. This education provides someone with the ability to take a certification exam in music therapy. Upon passing this exam, an individual can practice music therapy in a clinical setting and use the credential "MT-BC" after their name (American Music Therapy Association, 2019).

Music Therapy and Occupational Therapy

Only those who possess certification as a music therapist can perform music therapy. Music therapy can be performed in hospitals, nursing facilities, long-term care settings, hospice units, schools, outpatient clinics, or private practice settings. This modality is best used in a quiet, distraction-free environment. Music therapy can be performed during individual sessions or group therapy, depending on patient needs, preference, and the type of activity being implemented.

Music therapy cannot be completed as the main modality in a treatment session unless the occupational therapist holds the required certification. However, therapists may incorporate the use of music into occupational therapy treatment as a preparatory activity to encourage relaxation for engagement in functional tasks later or as background noise to improve performance during sessions. Music therapy can be combined with symptom management, emotion regulation, leisure exploration, play activities, and more.

CONSIDERATIONS FOR PRACTICE

Due to the risks associated with an unqualified professional providing music therapy to patients, therapists must implement this modality carefully and thoughtfully. Occupational therapists who wish to incorporate music into treatment can use many variations to prepare patients for other activities or to establish music as a hobby and healthy stress management tool. If the therapist wants their patient to play or make certain types of music, they should provide them with the appropriate materials (actual instruments or common objects used to create music). Patients should be given materials and a setting that are appropriate for their abilities (e.g., an area to sit while playing bongos). Therapists can choose whether patients need a semiprivate area or not based on whether they think the patient would benefit from a group activity or a secluded area where they can engage in personal discussions afterward.

Therapists may write music therapy–related goals in some of the following areas:

- Improving relaxation
- Establishing productive leisure
- Productively expressing emotions
- Regulating behaviors
- Sequencing activity steps
- Strengthening seated or standing activity tolerance
- Planning and appropriately using tools
- Increasing gross range of motion of the shoulder, elbow, or wrist
- Improving fine motor strength, motion, and coordination
- Enhancing core strength, stability, and head/neck control

CHAPTER 29

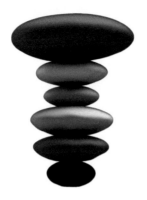

Neurolinguistic Programming

Neurolinguistic programming (NLP) is a modality that focuses on symbiotic communication by tapping into the unconscious mind. This technique uses a variety of methods to tap into the "language of your mind" to get the most out of life (Figure 29-1). NLP involves using your conscious mind as the goal setter of your life and the unconscious mind as the goal getter. Many people may experience the negative effects of their unconscious minds and this can stop them from functioning in certain ways. By channeling the unconscious mind using NLP, an individual can break certain habits and fully engage in daily life.

There is much more to communication than verbal expression, and these nonverbal communications are a foundational part of NLP theory. NLP helps modify an individual's inner communication to promote the breaking of bad habits and form positive function (Advanced Neurodynamics, 2015).

Ferri, B. *Complementary Health Approaches for Occupational Therapists* (pp. 143-146). © 2021 Taylor & Francis Group.

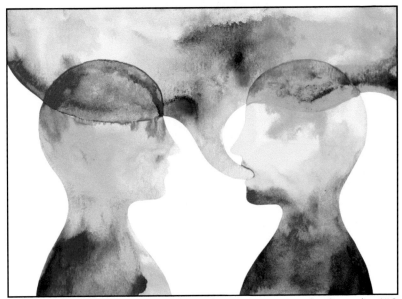

Figure 29-1. Knowing the language of the mind is an important part of understanding NLP. Benjavisa Ruangvaree Art/Shutterstock.com

BENEFITS

Anecdotal evidence suggests NLP is most beneficial for individuals with phobias, depression, anxiety, and self-limiting behaviors and thoughts. However, there is a lack of research proving NLP's efficacy for any purpose. One study showed NLP can be effective at reducing anxiety of individuals with claustrophobia who are undergoing magnetic resonance imaging (Bigley et al., 2010). Another study showed NLP is a brief and easy-to-use modality for individuals with phobias (Karunaratne, 2010). An additional study has shown NLP is more effective for short-term weight loss than a gourmet cooking group (Sorenson et al., 2011).

CONTRAINDICATIONS, PRECAUTIONS, AND SIDE EFFECTS

There are no known risks or contraindications associated with NLP. The effectiveness of NLP is partially based on an individual's interest in participating in NLP, as it involves consistent conscious participation and communicative engagement.

BASICS OF NEUROLINGUISTIC PROGRAMMING

Rapport: Building relationships with others and connecting through a combination of trust and body language is key in NLP. This can be built through understanding someone's preferences and accessing the visual cues a person gives off.

Sensory awareness: This trains someone to notice colors, smells, sounds, and sights that are quite different from those they are familiar with. This sensory input can then be used to calm the brain by paying attention to all that is around.

Outcome thinking: By connecting with the goal one has in mind, one can break out of a negative way of thinking. This can help people make informed decisions and choices that are best for their life situation.

Behavioral flexibility: Being able to change the way one does something after a period of realizing it does not work is paramount to accessing one's full potential. This flexibility helps everyone experience a fresh point of view and add new, more productive habits into their lifestyle (International Neurolinguistic Programming Center, 2018).

CREDENTIALING

A license is not required to practice NLP on patients. However, a certification and the associated training are recommended. This training gives the full picture of how NLP can help patients and allows for in-person implementation as practice. These trainings are available both in person and online, and vary in length and hours required (International Neurolinguistic Programming Center, 2018).

NEUROLINGUISTIC PROGRAMMING AND OCCUPATIONAL THERAPY

Any occupational therapy practice can incorporate NLP. A private practice or outpatient setting where there is ample space and an increased likelihood of a quiet, distraction-free environment is best for NLP. This modality is most appropriate for individual sessions, when used as a preparatory activity to encourage relaxation for engagement in functional tasks. This modality can be combined with lifestyle redesign, symptom management, social skills training, emotion regulation, vocational training, leisure exploration, and more.

CONSIDERATIONS FOR PRACTICE

Therapists should use NLP with patients in a private area where they feel comfortable discussing emotional events, personal insecurities, current relationship concerns, or past traumas with their therapist. Therapists need to have some prior knowledge about their patient's personal history, which they can obtain during the first session. Therapists who complete this evaluation will have data to inform their practice and allow them to help patients work through unhealthy habits, difficult emotions, or other personal matters. Therapists do not need additional tools or resources, aside from having experience with the NLP narrative to use with patients.

Therapists may write NLP-related goals in some of the following areas:

- Developing plans to use healthy, productive routines and habits to cope with any presenting concerns
- Building self-confidence and managing personal insecurities
- Understanding the mind-body connection and how it pertains to their life
- Incorporating the principles of NLP into a daily self-care routine
- Recognizing unhealthy behaviors and habits
- Improving communication skills
- Enhancing the quality of interpersonal relationships

CHAPTER 30

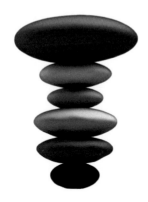

Orthomolecular Nutrition

Orthomolecular nutrition, or *orthomolecular medicine,* is the practice of providing the body with optimal amounts of natural substances in order to both prevent and address disease. Substances recommended include essential nutrients, such as proteins, carbohydrates, fats, oils, minerals, vitamins, and water, along with micronutrients (Figure 30-1). These substances are intended to encourage mental and physical health through diet and supplementation (Riordan Clinic, 2017).

BENEFITS

There is minimal research on orthomolecular nutrition, and much of the foundational background is from the 1970s. Studies that have been done are outdated, though they show some utility in certain circumstances.

Ferri, B. *Complementary Health Approaches for Occupational Therapists* (pp. 147-152).
© 2021 Taylor & Francis Group.

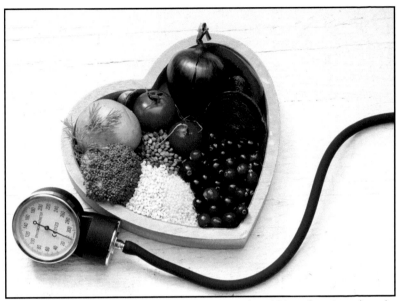

Figure 30-1. Orthomolecular nutrition can encourage the addition of nutrients through diet or other supplements. udra11/Shutterstock.com

A research study showed no benefit of orthomolecular supplementation in children with attention deficit hyperactivity disorder, with the only result being increases in serum transaminase levels of the children (Canadian Paediatric Society, 1990). This same study disproved the idea that megadoses of vitamin C could increase the quantity of white blood cells to improve upper respiratory infections. A course of vitamin A supplementation through a nutrition program reduced the risk of xerophthalmia, child mortality, and new Bitot's spots in developmentally disabled children. This study also showed higher compliance rates at a lower cost than alternate interventions, suggesting these types of programs are sustainable in the long term (Pant et al., 1996).

Other research studied the use of supplements, including vitamin C, vitamin E, coenzyme Q10, alpha-lipoic acid, chromium, l-carnitine, and quercetin. These supplements were found to benefit individuals with diabetes, cardiovascular disease, hypertension, heart failure, age-related cognitive and visual decline, and impaired immune function (Janson, 2006).

CONTRAINDICATIONS, PRECAUTIONS, AND SIDE EFFECTS

Major risks associated with orthomolecular nutrition are related to the concept of megadosing vitamins and minerals. Megadosing involves taking substantial quantities of dietary supplements and can result in toxicity, organ damage, and even death. While recommended daily doses of such substances have no associated risks, research should be done regarding safe amounts of any vitamin, mineral, or other supplement. Orthomolecular nutrition is not contraindicated with any population but should be supervised by a trained professional.

CREDENTIALING

Naturopathic physicians undergo significant training related to diet and nutrition and possess a certification and licensure to make specific recommendations. Naturopathic medical school consists of 4 years of educational content mixed with internships and practical experience. This can be completed after an undergraduate degree in a health-related field. The Association of Accredited Naturopathic Medical Colleges has accredited seven naturopathic medicine programs in the United States with hybrid courses consisting of some online training.

ORTHOMOLECULAR NUTRITION AND OCCUPATIONAL THERAPY

Only therapists who possess certification and licensure as a naturopathic physician can practice orthomolecular nutrition and naturopathic medicine. Occupational therapists are able to make standard diet recommendations to promote health, wellness, and general healing of the body. However, supplemental substances are not within occupational therapy's scope of practice.

Diet-related recommendations can be made as part of therapeutic education to supplement other types of wellness interventions. This modality can be combined with lifestyle redesign, symptom management, life skills training, self-care training, community integration, instrumental activities of daily living (like grocery shopping and cooking), and more.

Basics of Orthomolecular Nutrition

Calcium can be found in:

almonds	Brazil nuts	broccoli	cabbage
caviar	cheese	collards	dairy foods
dandelion leaves	dulse	figs	filberts
green leafy vegetables	kale	kelp	milk
molasses	mustard greens	oats	parsley
prunes	salmon	sardines	seafood
sesame seeds	shrimp	soybeans	tofu
turnip greens	yogurt		

Calcium helps clot blood, build muscle, and form strong bones, teeth, and gums. Calcium also helps keep regular heart rhythm, calms nerve transmissions, and prevents muscle cramps. Calcium helps break down fats and assists in protein structuring within the body.

Chloride can be found in:

celery	kelp	olives	sea salt
table salt	tomatoes		

Chloride assists with producing stomach acid and transmitting nerve impulses. Chloride regulates water, acids, and bases along with electrolytes. Chloride kills harmful micro-organisms within the stomach.

Iodine can be found in:

asparagus	chard	cod	garlic
haddock	herring	iodized salts	Irish moss
kelp	lima beans	lobster	mushrooms
oysters	salmon	sea salt	seafood
seaweed	sesame seeds	shrimp	soybeans
spinach	squash	sunflower seeds	turnip greens

Iodine helps proper thyroid function and fat metabolism, along with growth and energy. Iodine assists in carbohydrate absorption in the body. Iodine helps with hair, skin, tooth, and nail strength along with metabolism and protein synthesis.

(continued)

BASICS OF ORTHOMOLECULAR NUTRITION (CONTINUED)

Iron can be found in:

almonds	avocados	beans	beef
beets	blue cohosh	bran	brewer's yeast
broccoli	cashews	caviar	cheddar cheese
chickweed	cocoa	dates	devil's claw
dried fruit	dulse	eggs	garbanzo beans
green leafy vegetables	kelp	legumes	lentils
liver	millet	molasses	mullein
mussels	oysters	parsley	peaches
pears	pennyroyal	pistachios	potatoes
poultry	prunes	pumpkins	raisins
rice	seaweed	sesame seeds	soybeans
spinach	sunflower seeds	walnuts	wheat bran
wheat germ	whole grains		

Iron supplies blood with protein and copper, while assisting in oxygenation of red blood cells. Iron improves enzyme function and is stored in the liver, spleen, bone marrow, and blood.

Magnesium can be found in:

almonds	barley	blackstrap molasses	bluefish
brewer's yeast	buckwheat	carp	cocoa
cod	cottonseed	figs	flounder
garlic	green leafy vegetables	halibut	herring
Irish moss	kelp	licorice	lima beans
meat	mackerel	millet	molasses
nettle	nuts	oat straw	oats
peaches	peanut butter	peanuts	peas
perch	seafood	sesame seeds	shrimp
snails	soybeans	sunflower seeds	swordfish
tofu	wheat	wheat bran	wheat germ
whole grains			

Magnesium helps healthy heart function, converts blood sugar into energy, and builds strong bones and teeth. Magnesium is helpful in preventing strokes and fueling neuromuscular contractions (Riordan Clinic, 2017).

CONSIDERATIONS FOR PRACTICE

Therapists trained in orthomolecular nutrition do not need any tools to implement this modality. Therapists can use this modality with patients in a semi-private area where they can discuss current and future diet plans. Therapists need to educate their patients that this modality cannot diagnose or treat any medical conditions, rather orthomolecular nutrition can provide a healthier lifestyle to potentially prevent the development of health conditions. Therapists will need notebooks and pens in order to write out plans and health recommendations for their patients.

Therapists may write orthomolecular nutrition–related goals in some of the following areas:

- Recognizing unhealthy behaviors and habits
- Modifying diet in a way that supports a healthy lifestyle
- Creating an exercise plan to increase physical activity and lower bodily inflammation
- Using health recommendations daily as part of a self-care routine
- Developing plans to increase compliance with healthy, productive routines and habits
- Understanding the mind-body connection and how it pertains to their life

Chapter 31

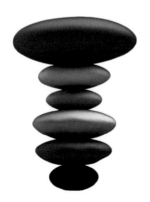

Progressive Muscle Relaxation

Progressive muscle relaxation (PMR) is a modality that uses the intermittent tensing and relaxing of muscles to elicit a bodily feeling of flexibility and calmness of the mind. This technique, when practiced regularly, is meant to bring awareness to tense muscles and what the body associates with tense muscles. This is intended to ease the frequency and intensity of muscle tension while helping to regulate the body's natural state. PMR can be practiced using an audio script, when led by an instructor or when following a set of instructions. To achieve the maximum effect, complete this practice in a place where you are comfortable and will not be interrupted (Figure 31-1).

Analyses of functional magnetic resonance imaging showed PMR decreased activity in the superior frontal gyrus, inferior frontal gyrus, and posterior cingulate cortex in 11 participants. Further analysis showed a relationship between activity in the putamen, anterior cingulate cortex, and insula (Kobayashi & Koitabashi, 2016).

The superior and inferior frontal gyri control sustained attention, working memory, and language processing, among other functions. The

Ferri, B. *Complementary Health Approaches
for Occupational Therapists* (pp. 153-156).
© 2021 Taylor & Francis Group.

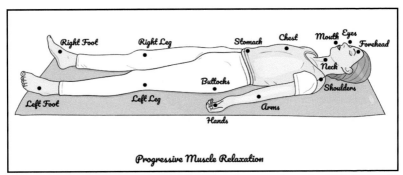

Figure 31-1. These are the main parts of the body to focus on when using PMR. dityazemli/ Shutterstock.com

cingulate cortex and insula govern emotion formation and regulation, along with processing, learning, and memory. The putamen assists in coordination and movement. Each of these functions is typically impacted by acute or chronic stress, making the brain activity created by PMR effective at relieving both mental and bodily discomfort (Kobayashi & Koitabashi, 2016).

BENEFITS

One research study showed PMR was effective in decreasing fatigue levels and improving subjective sleep quality and sleep duration of individuals with chronic obstructive pulmonary disease. This study showed PMR did not have an impact in global sleep quality (Seyedi Chegeni et al., 2018). Another study showed abbreviated PMR decreased cortisol levels and subjective stress levels in college students for one week (Chellew et al., 2015).

Another study showed PMR was effective in lowering scores related to apathy, irritability, and neuropsychiatric symptoms of group home residents with dementia symptoms. Significant improvements were also made in the outcome scores of interest, volition, social relationships, and activity of daily living participation (Ikemata & Momose, 2017).

CONTRAINDICATIONS, PRECAUTIONS, AND SIDE EFFECTS

There are no risks associated with PMR. PMR is contraindicated for those individuals with high blood pressure, any cardiovascular disease, or recent cardiac surgery.

BASICS OF PROGRESSIVE MUSCLE RELAXATION

PMR is best practiced in a comfortable position and in a quiet space free of distractions. Some people choose to start at the muscles located at the top of the body (e.g., the face) and work their way down to those at the bottom (e.g., the toes). However, this is dependent on personal preference and whether you are using a script. You can follow this set of instructions when using the chart below.

1. Breathe in and firmly, but not painfully, tense the first muscle group. Hold for 4 to 10 seconds.
2. Breathe out and completely relax the muscle group. Complete relaxation rather than gradual relaxation is recommended.
3. Relax for 10 to 20 seconds before moving to the next muscle group. Notice how your muscles feel when they are relaxed and how they feel when they are tense.
4. Repeat as needed for relaxation effect.
   - Make fists with both hands
   - Fully flex both wrists, then fully extend them
   - Bend elbows, make two fists, and flex biceps
   - Shrug your shoulders as close to your ears as you can
   - Wrinkle your forehead and arch your eyebrows
   - Squeeze your eyes closed tightly
   - Make the biggest smile you can
   - Squeeze your lips together while not moving the rest of your face
   - Lean back and press your head into the surface behind it
   - Squeeze your chin while trying to touch it to your chest
   - Hold a deep breath for 5 to 10 seconds
   - Arch your back away from the surface it is against
   - Sharply inhale and draw your stomach in toward your spine
   - Clench your buttocks together tightly
   - Squeeze your thighs together
   - Point your toes up and down, clenching in each direction (University of Michigan Medicine, 2018)

CREDENTIALING

There is no license or certification required to practice PMR. There is also no regulatory body governing the credentialing or practice of PMR. There are varying online training courses to provide further education in PMR techniques and how it can be applied to practice.

PROGRESSIVE MUSCLE RELAXATION AND OCCUPATIONAL THERAPY

Any occupational therapy practice can incorporate PMR. A private practice or outpatient setting where there is ample space and an increased likelihood of a quiet, distraction-free environment is best for PMR.

Therapists may incorporate the use of PMR into occupational therapy treatment as a preparatory activity to promote improved bodily flexibility, decreased muscle tension, and encourage relaxation for engagement in functional tasks. This modality can be implemented during individual sessions or during group therapy, depending on location and patient needs. PMR can be combined with symptom management, emotion regulation, leisure exploration, self-care training, and more.

CONSIDERATIONS FOR PRACTICE

Therapists can guide patients through PMR in a semiprivate setting, but this modality can also work in a standard therapy setting with little space. Patients should ideally have a place to sit, and therapists can provide amenities to increase their relaxation, such as blankets, essential oils, and comfortable seating.

Therapists can easily guide patients through PMR without a script, but some therapists may wish to follow a script to target certain muscles or parts of the body.

Therapists may write PMR-related goals in some of the following areas:

- Lowering pain levels
- Tracking symptoms before and after PMR
- Enhancing relaxation
- Practicing mindfulness
- Improving body awareness
- Understanding the mind-body connection and how it pertains to their life
- Incorporating PMR into a daily self-care routine

CHAPTER 32

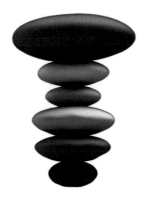

Qigong

Qigong is a mind-body modality that involves the use of certain postures and slow, gentle motions, along with concentration, awareness, and even breathing. Qigong has roots in Traditional Chinese Medicine and uses the idea of moving energy, or *qi*, to achieve wellness and relief from pain (Figure 32-1). The open flow of energy through the meridians intends to improve connection and communication with the Earth's life force. Qigong's main focus is on eliminating energy deficiencies within the body and moving energy stagnations in order to prevent chronic illness and pain (National Qigong Association, n.d.).

Ferri, B. *Complementary Health Approaches*
for Occupational Therapists (pp. 157-161).
© 2021 Taylor & Francis Group.

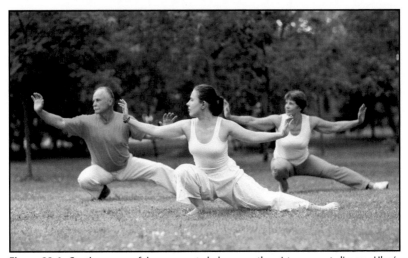

Figure 32-1. Gentle, purposeful movements help move the qi to prevent disease. Ulza/ Shutterstock.com

BENEFITS

Anecdotal evidence suggests the movement associated with qigong warms tendons, ligaments, and muscles; tonifies organs and muscle tissue; and improves whole body circulation. Anecdotal evidence also states qigong can assist with high blood pressure, chronic pain, anxiety, and depression.

One research study showed qigong was effective in lowering weight, waist circumference, insulin resistance, and fasting blood insulin, while increasing leg strength of individuals with diabetes (Liu et al., 2011). Another study showed a combination of tai chi and qigong significantly improved hypertension, fasting blood glucose levels, body mass index, and levels of homeostasis (Lauche et al., 2017).

Another study combining qigong and tai chi significantly improved motor coordination, balance, depressive symptoms, and quality of life while decreasing scores on Timed Up and Go and risk of falls (Song et al., 2017). Another study showed that individuals who participated in qigong regularly experienced improved stress levels, resiliency, feelings of empowerment, sleep quality, and physical function in wounded military members (Reb et al., 2017).

BASICS OF QIGONG

Self-massage: Warm your eyes. Rub your palms together and then place them against your eyes for 5 seconds. Repeat three times. Roll your eyes. Start by looking up and then circle 10 times clockwise and 10 times counterclockwise. Hold a pen at arm's length and focus on it. Slowly bring the pen closer until it is inches from your nose. Slowly move it back, remaining focused on the pen. Repeat 10 times total. Massage your temples. Using your thumbs, massage your temples in small circles, 20 times one way and 20 times the other way. Repeat just above the nose at the forehead and again below each eye.

First mindful alignment: Sit, stand, or lie outstretched. Visualize a string lifting your head into the heavens. Visualize a connection between your sacrum and the earth. Feel the lift and pull open the body and fill it with life-force energy. Aligning the spine creates spaces between the vertebrae and releases compression on the nerves that may cause pain or discomfort. Adjusting your posture allows for the space your organs need to function optimally and also optimizes the inner flow of blood and lymph.

Second mindful alignment: Inhale slowly through your nose, hold your breath for a count of 3. Allow your breaths to be deep and slow. On the exhalation, relax even more.

Third mindful alignment: For as long as possible, focus your mind on something simple. This can be clouds, water, waves, a forest, a beach, a meadow, or anything. Let go of all thoughts. Simply be mindful, noticing where you are, what you are doing, and what you are sensing (Qigong Institute, 2019).

CONTRAINDICATIONS, PRECAUTIONS, AND SIDE EFFECTS

There are no risks or side effects associated with qigong. Due to traditional qigong being completed in standing, this modality is contraindicated for those individuals who have severely or moderately impaired mobility and those who do not have the upper extremity range of motion to participate. There are portions of qigong that may be modified for a sitting population and this can be utilized for certain patients who may benefit from qigong.

Credentialing

There is no license required to perform qigong. Individuals wishing to pursue certification can do so from the National Qigong Association. Level one qigong instructor certification consists of 200 hours of training; level two qigong instructor certification consists of 350 hours of training; and level three qigong instructor certification consists of 500 hours of training (National Qigong Association, n.d.).

Qigong and Occupational Therapy

Any occupational therapy practice can incorporate qigong if it is determined to be safe for the patient. Qigong can be completed in a hospital, nursing facility, school, long-term care unit, outpatient clinic, private practice, or any other setting where there is ample space and an increased likelihood of a quiet, distraction-free environment.

Therapists may incorporate the use of qigong into occupational therapy treatment as a preparatory activity to encourage relaxation for engagement in functional tasks later, or as a part of therapeutic exercise to improve balance, coordination, range of motion, strength, and more. Qigong can be combined with lifestyle redesign, symptom management, emotion regulation, self-care training, life skills, social skills, leisure exploration, and more.

Considerations for Practice

This modality does not require the use of any equipment. Therapists should ideally practice qigong with patients in a quiet space with room for movement, but patients can easily practice this modality in a patient exam room. Individuals would benefit from therapists serving as visual models for the qigong sequence or following a visual model from a video. Therapists who are advanced in their own qigong practice can guide patients through this modality without a script or prior preparation. However, some therapists may need patients to follow a video while providing patients with feedback on their form and posture throughout the process. Therapists should have prior knowledge of a patient's medical history and presenting concerns so they can prepare specific sequences to improve symptoms and avoid aggravating other injuries or medical conditions.

Therapists may write qigong-related goals in some of the following areas:
- Enhancing relaxation and mindfulness
- Improving range of motion
- Increasing endurance
- Enhancing strength and activity tolerance
- Following directions
- Decreasing pain levels
- Increasing independence in transfers and functional mobility
- Utilizing safety awareness and judgment
- Managing uncomfortable emotions, such as sadness, irritability, or trauma-related concerns
- Becoming independent in the use of qigong in their daily self-care routine
- Increasing education regarding the mind-body connection
- Improving balance and coordination
- Remembering the qigong sequence independently

CHAPTER 33

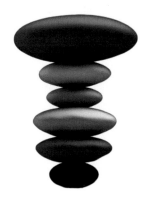

Reflexology

Reflexology is a modality that involves the application of pressure to points on the hands or feet (Figure 33-1). The idea behind reflexology is similar to that of acupuncture, acupressure, and auriculotherapy in that each point corresponds with a particular point in the body. Manipulation of these points is intended to bring relief from multiple symptoms.

The practice of reflexology works with the central nervous system by sending nerve impulses from the extremities throughout the body. These nerve impulses signal the body to adjust levels of tension, intended to bring internal organs to a level of optimum functioning, increase blood flow, and speed up waste removal. Reflexology also works with the gate theory by acting on the sensory processes that elicit the chronic pain response.

Ferri, B. *Complementary Health Approaches for Occupational Therapists* (pp. 163-166). © 2021 Taylor & Francis Group.

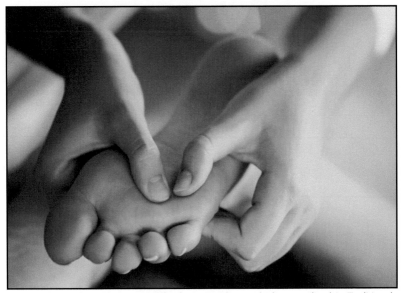

Figure 33-1. Reflexology zones differ from meridians, which are utilized in Traditional Chinese Medicine–based modalities. Africa Studio/Shutterstock.com

The feet are divided into 10 zones that each correspond to areas all over the body. These zones are intended to have a direct connection with each bodily system, making them able to relieve associated symptoms. While reflexology uses some of the same principles and foundations as acupuncture, reflexology zones are not the same as the meridians from acupuncture or Traditional Chinese Medicine (University of Minnesota, 2016).

Benefits

Anecdotal evidence suggests reflexology is effective in addressing conditions, such as anxiety, asthma, cancer, cardiovascular disease, migraines, kidney disorders, premenstrual syndrome, and sinusitis.

Research shows reflexology decreases pain, intensity, duration, and anxiety related to active labor (Moghimi-Hanjani et al., 2015). Another study indicates reflexology lowers pain levels of women with breast cancer, while increasing functional participation and general health condition (Ozdelikara & Tan, 2017). Reflexology has been proven to decrease dyspnea and fatigue in patients with chronic obstructive pulmonary disease (Polat & Erguney, 2017). A protocol of reflexology also elicited a high degree of sleep quality, indicating subjectively increased levels of relaxation (Esmel-Esmel et al., 2017).

CONTRAINDICATIONS, PRECAUTIONS, AND SIDE EFFECTS

There are no risks associated with the practice of reflexology. Reflexology is contraindicated for patients at risk for blood clots, patients with foot injuries or open wounds, as well as women who are pregnant. Bodily manipulation can worsen foot injuries, move existing clots to the brain or heart, and cause infection to open wounds.

CREDENTIALING

Licenses in reflexology are only available in North Dakota and Tennessee. Washington requires a certification in reflexology in order to practice. Certifications are recommended and available in all other states to ensure regulated practice and standard procedures. The typical reflexology course consists of 15 to 30 hours of educational content and practical experience. Massage therapy schools also offer continuing education courses in reflexology (University of Minnesota, 2016).

REFLEXOLOGY AND OCCUPATIONAL THERAPY

Reflexology can only be practiced by those who possess certification and licensure, in the appropriate states. Therapists wishing to practice reflexology in a state where a license is not available are encouraged to complete a certification and associated training program.

Reflexology can be completed in hospitals, nursing facilities, long term care units, schools, outpatient clinics, or private practices. This modality can be completed during individual sessions or group therapy. Reflexology can be performed as the main modality to enhance health and wellness in patients or as a preparatory activity to encourage relaxation for engagement in functional tasks. Reflexology can be combined with lifestyle redesign, symptom management, emotion regulation, self-care training, and more.

CONSIDERATIONS FOR PRACTICE

This modality does not require the use of any equipment. Therapists should ideally implement reflexology in a quiet space, but there is no need for individuals to be in a large, spacious area. Reflexology requires therapists to work on a patient's feet, so they must remove shoes and socks to provide this modality. As therapists instruct patients how to complete this modality outside of therapy sessions, individuals would benefit from therapist demonstration or visual models via videos or images. Therapists who have prior knowledge of a patient's main areas of concern can prepare specific sequences or routines that would benefit patients. However, therapists who have more experience in reflexology can devise patient routines on the spot based on issues that a patient reports or is currently demonstrating.

Therapists may write reflexology-related goals in some of the following areas:

- Becoming independent in the use of reflexology as a stress management tool
- Increasing education regarding the mind-body connection
- Improving relaxation
- Enhancing sleep hygiene
- Remembering the sequence for a certain number of reflexology points
- Fine-tuning their force modulation to elicit the optimal response from each reflexology point
- Incorporating reflexology into a daily self-care routine

CHAPTER 34

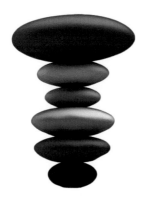

Reiki

Reiki is a form of energy medicine meant to promote healing, relaxation, and stress reduction. This subtle form of energy medicine uses occasional light touch, with the majority of the focus on the laying of hands immediately above the body to assist with the movement of energy (Figure 34-1). This modality focuses on bodily life force, as low bodily life force is what reiki practitioners believe to be the cause of sickness and stress. High bodily life force is intended to cause happiness and health.

Reiki can be performed sitting or on a massage table. However, unlike massage, no articles of clothing are removed. A reiki practitioner will ask the individual if they have any discomfort or physical and emotional complaints. They will then practice the standard hand positions and begin at the head or toes, providing the individual with a slight warming sensation or relaxation. Reiki can also be completed long-distance by experienced practitioners in the form of prayer and sending of energy (The International Center for Reiki Training, 2019).

Ferri, B. *Complementary Health Approaches for Occupational Therapists* (pp. 167-170).
© 2021 Taylor & Francis Group.

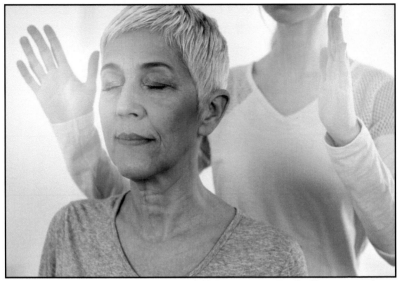

Figure 34-1. As a form of energy medicine, reiki aims to manipulate bodily energy without the use of touch. Albina Glisic/Shutterstock.com

BENEFITS

Anecdotal evidence suggests reiki is effective in relieving pain, anxiety, and depression. However, there is minimal research supporting reiki for this purpose. One research study showed neither reiki nor therapeutic touch had any impact on the pain levels of individuals with fibromyalgia (Assefi et al., 2008). Another research study showed reiki was effective in decreasing pain and anxiety in cancer patients along with community-dwelling adults (Thrane & Cohen, 2015).

Research has also shown reiki and therapeutic touch are somewhat effective in reducing pain, nausea, anxiety, and fatigue along with raising life quality (Tabatabaee et al., 2016). Another study showed variable results on the effectiveness of reiki and therapeutic touch on acute wounds. Out of four participants, two showed significantly faster and more effective healing, one showed significantly worse wound healing, and another showed no significant differences (O'Mathuna, 2016). An additional study showed reiki had no significant impact on reducing oral pain in a pediatric population (Kundu et al., 2015).

CONTRAINDICATIONS, PRECAUTIONS, AND SIDE EFFECTS

There are no risks associated with reiki. Due to the light touch or simple hovering of the hands above the body, there is no manipulation as with other therapeutic touch or manual modalities. Therefore, there are also no contraindications associated with reiki.

CREDENTIALING

No license is required to practice reiki. Certifications are available online and in-person and are recommended to receive the proper training. Level one reiki certification can be obtained in a one-weekend intensive course. Those seeking further training can receive two additional levels in order to become a reiki master, also known as the highest level of certification.

REIKI AND OCCUPATIONAL THERAPY

Any occupational therapist can incorporate reiki without a certification or extensive training. A private practice or outpatient setting where there is ample space and an increased likelihood of a quiet, distraction-free environment is best for reiki.

Therapists may incorporate the use of reiki into occupational therapy treatment as a preparatory activity to encourage relaxation and decrease pain for engagement in functional tasks. Reiki can be combined with lifestyle redesign, symptom management, emotion regulation, self-care training, life skills, leisure exploration, and more.

CONSIDERATIONS FOR PRACTICE

Therapists do not need any tools or equipment to guide patients through reiki. Therapists would benefit from providing patients with a quiet, private room where both parties can focus and feel comfortable during the process. Patients receiving reiki often need to lay down or remain seated, so therapists should have a cushioned padded treatment table or mat with blankets to make patients comfortable. While full reiki sessions require patients to receive energy from another person (therapist to patient), there are short reiki sequences that therapists can teach patients to elicit similar benefits outside of therapy sessions. Therapists can give patients visual images or videos for reference to help them complete these sequences in between sessions as part of their self-care routine.

Therapists may write reiki-related goals in some of the following areas:

- Understanding the mind-body connection and how it pertains to their life
- Becoming independent in the use of some reiki techniques as a stress management tool
- Increasing education regarding the mind-body connection
- Enhancing relaxation
- Practicing mindfulness
- Improving sleep hygiene
- Managing uncomfortable emotions
- Demonstrating improved motivation and general engagement in therapy or other occupations
- Remembering the steps for the reiki sequence
- Incorporating reiki into a daily self-care routine

CHAPTER 35

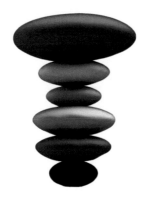

Tai Chi

Tai chi is a mind-body modality that involves self-movement of energy, gentle physical exercise with stretching, and rhythmic breathing (Figure 35-1). This is meant to reduce stress, encourage relaxation, and enhance the mind-body connection. Tai chi was originally developed for self-defense, and those who take advanced training can use it for that purpose. Tai chi can be thought of as meditation in slow motion, due to its rhythmic and gentle movements. Tai chi is low impact, placing low stress on the muscles and joints. One of the main focuses of tai chi is making each motion flow seamlessly into the next without a pause. This places the body in constant motion, assisting in the balancing of energy.

BENEFITS

Anecdotal evidence suggests tai chi is effective in decreasing stress, anxiety, and depression, while improving mood, aerobic capacity, energy, flexibility, and muscle strength. One research study showed tai chi and qigong were of average effectiveness in decreasing blood pressure, fasting

Ferri, B. *Complementary Health Approaches for Occupational Therapists* (pp. 171-174). © 2021 Taylor & Francis Group.

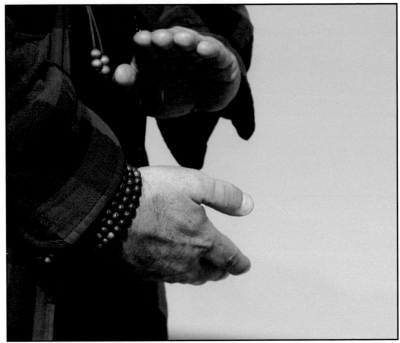

Figure 35-1. Forming an energy ball with the hands is common in tai chi and is also part of similar Eastern practices, such as qigong. Joanne Laskey/Shutterstock.com

blood glucose, and body mass index of individuals with hypertension, hyperlipidemia, diabetes, and obesity (Lauche et al., 2017).

Another study showed regular practice of tai chi improved circulation in the lower extremities, placed major depressive disorder in remission, lowered blood pressure, improved standing balance, and improved cognitive function in older adults (Lan et al., 2013). Research also shows tai chi is more effective in improving generalized levels of fatigue than conventional therapies. This same study showed tai chi positively impacted cancer-related fatigue levels, while improving sleep patterns, depressive symptoms, and overall vitality in a different set of participants (Xiang et al., 2017).

Additional research showed tai chi had a greater impact on anxiety, self-efficacy, and coping of individuals with fibromyalgia than aerobic exercise (Wang et al., 2018). One study showed tai chi caused significant gain in mental-attentional capacity, attentional inhibition, fluid intelligence measure, and attentional balance of participants (Kim et al., 2016).

CONTRAINDICATIONS, PRECAUTIONS, AND SIDE EFFECTS

There are no risks associated with tai chi. Due to the gentle movements and the ability for tai chi to be modified for populations with more severe mobility impairments, there is a minimal fall risk for patients who participate. There are also no contraindications associated with tai chi.

CREDENTIALING

There is no license required to practice tai chi. Certifications are available online and in-person and are recommended to receive the proper training. Certification can be obtained after 150 hours of educational content and hands-on experience. Individuals may then seek certification through the American Tai Chi and Qigong Association. Those who have received training far above the minimum requirement while teaching in the community can become teaching assistants and begin their own classes (American Tai Chi and Qigong Association, 2010).

TAI CHI AND OCCUPATIONAL THERAPY

Occupational therapists can incorporate tai chi into any practice without a certification or extensive training. Tai chi can be performed in hospitals, nursing facilities, schools, long-term care units, outpatient clinics, or private practice. It is best suited in a place with ample space and an increased likelihood of a quiet, distraction-free environment.

Therapists may incorporate the use of tai chi into occupational therapy treatment as a preparatory activity to improve balance, coordination, and range of motion, and to encourage relaxation and pain relief for engagement in functional tasks. This modality can be combined with lifestyle redesign, symptom management, emotion regulation, social skills training, self-care training, leisure exploration, and more.

CONSIDERATIONS FOR PRACTICE

This modality does not require the use of any equipment. Therapists should ideally practice tai chi with patients in a quiet space with room for movement, but patients can easily practice this modality in a patient exam room. Individuals would benefit from therapists serving as visual models for the tai chi sequence or following a visual model from a video. Therapists who are advanced in their own tai chi practice can guide patients through this modality without a script or prior preparation. However, some therapists may need patients to follow a video while providing patients with feedback on their form and posture throughout the process. Therapists should have prior knowledge of a patient's medical history and presenting concerns so they can prepare specific sequences to improve symptoms and avoid aggravating other injuries or medical conditions.

Therapists may write tai chi–related goals in some of the following areas:

- Enhancing strength and activity tolerance
- Following directions
- Decreasing pain levels
- Increasing independence in transfers and functional mobility
- Enhancing relaxation and mindfulness
- Improving range of motion
- Increasing endurance
- Utilizing safety awareness and judgment
- Managing uncomfortable emotions, such as sadness, irritability, or trauma-related concerns
- Becoming independent in the use of tai chi in their daily self-care routine
- Increasing education regarding the mind-body connection
- Improving balance and coordination
- Remembering the tai chi sequence independently

CHAPTER 36

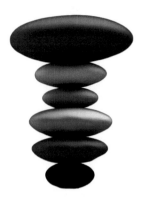

Yoga

Yoga is a modality with strong roots in Indian and Ayurvedic medicine practices. Yoga originated as a primarily spiritual practice. This has evolved into a mind-body practice that uses posture, form, breath work, and meditation to increase physical and mental well-being (Figure 36-1). There are several forms of yoga and all have varying benefits and postures. The most common type of yoga in the United States is hatha yoga, with associated styles, such as vini, bikram, and kundalini. The major principles of yoga are postures (called *asanas*), breath work (called *pranayama*), and meditation (called *dyana*) (National Center for Complementary and Integrative Health, 2018d).

BENEFITS

Anecdotal evidence suggests yoga is effective in reducing symptoms associated with anxiety, depressive disorders, and post-traumatic stress disorder. Research shows yoga caused significant improvements in mental manipulation, letter-number sequencing, and mindfulness

Ferri, B. *Complementary Health Approaches for Occupational Therapists* (pp. 175-178).

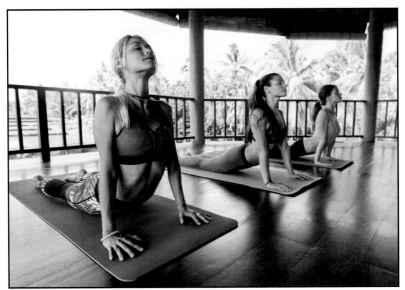

Figure 36-1. In recent years, yoga has become a popular mind-body activity. Jacob Lund/ Shutterstock.com

of older adults (Brunner et al., 2017). Another study showed yoga caused a significant increase in the psychological well-being of healthy adults when compared to no intervention (Hendriks et al., 2017).

Research showed women with prenatal depression showed significantly decreased levels of depression after practicing integrated yoga, including breath work, meditation, or relaxation techniques. This compared to only slightly lower levels of depression in women who practiced exercise-based yoga (Gong et al., 2015).

Another study compared the benefits of three separate groups completing pilates, yoga, and isometric exercise along with conventional therapy on individuals with chronic neck pain. All groups demonstrated improvements in levels of pain, disability, depression, and quality of life. Only the group who participated in pilates demonstrated an increase in muscle thickness (Ulug et al., 2018).

Another study showed military veterans with lower back pain had greater improvements in levels of health disability and pain intensity than participants who received delayed intervention. Participants also demonstrated a decrease in the use of opioid medications as a result of the intervention (Groessl et al., 2017).

Contraindications, Precautions, and Side Effects

Risks of yoga include spraining or straining muscles or joints if practiced incorrectly. Certain yoga poses are contraindicated for pregnant women, older adults, or patients with severe dyspnea or osteoporosis, due to the risk of injury.

Hot yoga, also known as *bikram yoga*, involves the use of a sauna that places individuals at risk for overheating and dehydrating if they do not take appropriate precautions. These patients must consult their doctor before participating. Those who practice bikram yoga should be sure to drink plenty of fluids and be mindful of symptoms, such as dizziness, excess fatigue, or lack of coordination. Saunas should not be used for extended periods of time.

The practice of yoga postures involving inversions, twisting upside-down, is contraindicated in patients with glaucoma. As glaucoma is a pressure-related disorder, upside-down positions could cause an increase in blood pressure in the facial region, causing temporary loss of vision or blindness.

Credentialing

There is no licensure for yoga; however, certification is required to teach yoga classes in isolation. The minimum requirement for certification is 200 hours of educational content and hands-on training. Those interested in further training can also obtain a 500-hour certification that can be combined with specializations. Educational content consists of anatomy and physiology, yoga principles, philosophy, postures, and breath work (Yoga Alliance, 2018).

Yoga and Occupational Therapy

The basics of yoga can easily be incorporated into any therapy session, if the individual would benefit from it. Yoga can be performed in hospitals, nursing facilities, long-term care units, schools, outpatient clinics, and private practices. A quiet area with ample space that allows for as little distractions as possible is recommended for yoga. Floor yoga will also require mats, blocks, straps, and pillows. However, chair yoga can be completed with simply a bench, chair, or other seating option. Yoga can be completed during individual sessions or during group therapy, depending on patient needs, location, and available materials.

Yoga can be completed as a therapeutic exercise to improve balance, coordination, flexibility, range of motion, and strength. Yoga can also be used as a preparatory activity to encourage relaxation and pain relief to improve engagement in functional tasks. Yoga can be combined with lifestyle redesign, symptom management, emotion regulation, life skills, leisure exploration, social skills training, community integration, and more.

Considerations for Practice

While most yoga simply requires a mat, many therapists require or allow patients to choose whether they want to use blocks and straps as well. Patients can receive deeper stretches by using these additional tools. Therapists working with an older or otherwise frail population who is at risk for falls may choose to lead patients in modified chair yoga, where all poses are in a seated position. Therapists should ideally practice yoga with patients in a quiet, open space to allow for enough focus and room for movement. Patients with any amount of experience in yoga would benefit from therapists serving as visual models for yoga sequences. Therapists who are advanced in their own yoga practice can guide patients through this modality without prior preparation. However, some therapists may need patients to follow a video while providing patients with feedback on their form and posture throughout the process. Therapists should provide patients with continual feedback regarding their posture, positioning, and form throughout their yoga practice. Therapists should have prior knowledge of a patient's medical history and presenting concerns so they can prepare specific sequences to improve symptoms and avoid aggravating other injuries or medical conditions.

Therapists may write yoga-related goals in some of the following areas:

- Increasing independence in transfers and functional mobility
- Enhancing relaxation and mindfulness
- Improving range of motion
- Increasing endurance
- Utilizing safety awareness and judgment
- Enhancing strength and activity tolerance
- Following directions
- Decreasing pain levels
- Managing uncomfortable emotions, such as sadness, irritability, or trauma-related concerns
- Becoming independent in the use of yoga in their daily self-care routine
- Increasing education regarding the mind-body connection
- Improving balance and coordination
- Remembering the yoga sequence independently

CHAPTER 37

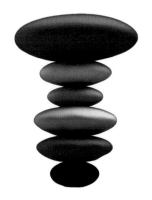

In Summary

It is your ethical responsibility as a therapist to educate the patient on any potential hazards or risks of the modalities you are aware of. If needed, it is necessary to modify your treatment plan accordingly for the safety of the patient.

As always, it is important to document all of this information from a patient to ensure the occupational therapist is keeping safety first and intending to do no harm. Occupational therapists should also document the counsel and education provided to patients regarding all modalities and conditions. Health education is one of the most important ways occupational therapists can assist patients in achieving function and wellness. These risks should be taken seriously, and all potential hazards or contraindications should be weighed carefully before implementing any modalities or informing a patient of their benefits.

CHAPTER 38

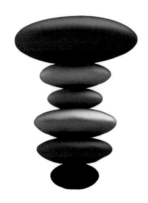

Resources

Academy for Guided Imagery
30765 CA-1
Suite 355
Malibu, CA 90265
Website: http://acadgi.com

American Art Therapy Association
4875 Eisenhower Avenue
Suite 240
Alexandria, VA 22304
Website: https://arttherapy.org

Ferri, B. *Complementary Health Approaches for Occupational Therapists* (pp. 181-185). © 2021 Taylor & Francis Group.

American Association of Drugless Practitioners
2200 Market Street
Suite 803
Galveston, TX 77550
Website: https://aadp.net

American Chiropractic Association
1701 Clarendon Boulevard
Suite 200
Arlington, VA 22209
Website: https://www.acatoday.org

American Herbalists Guild
P.O. Box 3076
Asheville, NC 28802
Website: https://www.americanherbalistsguild.com

American Music Therapy Association
8455 Colesville Road
Suite 1000
Silver Spring, MD 20910
Website: https://www.musictherapy.org

American Society of Clinical Hypnosis
140 N. Bloomingdale Road
Bloomingdale, IL 60108
Website: https://www.asch.net

American Tai Chi and Qigong Association
2465 J-17 Centreville Road
Suite 150
Herndon, VA 20171
Website: http://www.americantaichi.org

Animal Assisted Therapy Programs of Colorado
7275 Kipling Street
Arvada, CO 80005
Website: https://www.animalassistedtherapyprograms.org

Animal Behavior Institute, Inc.
4711 Hope Valley Road
Suite 4F-332
Durham, NC 27707
Website: https://www.animaledu.com

Aquatic Therapy and Rehabilitation Institute, Inc.
6602 Chestnut Circle
Naples, FL 34109
Website: http://www.atri.org

Association of Accredited Naturopathic Medical Colleges
1717 K Street NW
Suite 900
Washington, DC 20006
Website: https://aanmc.org

Auriculotherapy Certification Institute
8033 Sunset Boulevard
PMB 270
Los Angeles, CA, 90046
Website: https://www.auriculotherapy.org

Bach Original Flower Remedies Education
21 High Street
Suite 302
North Andover, MA 01845
Website: https://www.bachremedies.com/en-us/practitioners/
    how-to-become-a-practitioner

Biofeedback Certification International Alliance
5310 Ward Road
Suite 201
Arvada, CO 80002
Website: https://www.bcia.org

Board of Advanced Natural Health Sciences
Website: https://www.banhs.org

Eye Movement Desensitization and Reprocessing International Association
5806 Mesa Drive
Suite 360
Austin, TX 78731
Website: https://www.emdria.org

International Centre for Excellence in Emotionally Focused Therapy
201-1869 Carling Avenue
Ottawa, ON, Canada K2A 1C1
Website: https://iceeft.com/road-to-certification

International Iridology Practitioners Association
9 Office Park Circle
Suite 201
Mountain Brook, AL 35223
Website: https://www.iridologyassn.org

International Neurolinguistic Programming Center
41593 Winchester Road
Suite 200
Temecula, CA 92590
Website: https://inlpcenter.org

National Association for Holistic Aromatherapy
6000 S 5th Avenue
Pocatello, ID 83204
Website: https://naha.org

National Certification Board for Therapeutic Massage and Bodywork
1333 Burr Ridge Parkway
Suite 200
Burr Ridge, IL 60527
Website: https://www.ncbtmb.org

**National Certification Commission for Acupuncture
   and Oriental Medicine**
2025 M Street NW
Suite 800
Washington, DC 20036
Website: https://www.nccaom.org

National Qigong Association
P.O. Box 270065
St. Paul, MN 55127
Website: https://www.nqa.org

Upledger Institute International
11211 Prosperity Farms Road
Suite D325
Palm Beach Gardens, FL 33410
Website: https://www.upledger.com

Yoga Alliance
1560 Wilson Boulevard
Suite 700
Arlington, VA 22209
Website: https://www.yogaalliance.org

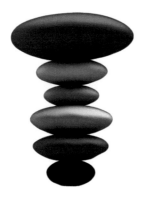

References

Acupuncture and Massage College. (2017). Eight principles of diagnosis in Traditional Chinese Medicine. (2017). Retrieved from https://www.amcollege.edu/blog/eight-principles-of-diagnosis-in-tcm

Advanced Neurodynamics. (2015). What is NLP. Retrieved from http://www.nlp.com/what-is-nlp/

Aguilar, B. A. (2017). The efficacy of art therapy in pediatric oncology patients: An integrative literature review. *Journal of Pediatric Nursing, 36,* 173-178. https://doi.org/10.1016/j.pedn.2017.06.015

Alvarez, M. J., Fernandez, D., Gomez-Salgado, J., Rodriguez-Gonzalez, D., Roson, M., & Lapena, S. (2017). The effects of massage therapy in hospitalized preterm neonates: A systematic review. *International Journal of Nursing Studies, 69,* 119-136. https://doi.org/10.1016/j.ijnurstu.2017.02.009

American Addiction Centers. (2018). Understanding the benefits of animal-assisted therapies. Retrieved from https://americanaddictioncenters.org/therapy-treatment/animal-assisted

American Art Therapy Association. (2013). What is art therapy? Retrieved from http://www.arttherapy.org/upload/whatisarttherapy.pdf

American Chiropractic Association. (2019). Chiropractic qualifications. Retrieved from https://www.acatoday.org/Patients/Why-Choose-Chiropractic/Chiropractic-Qualifications

Ferri, B. *Complementary Health Approaches for Occupational Therapists* (pp. 187-199). © 2021 Taylor & Francis Group.

American Kennel Club. (2015). Training your dog to be a therapy dog. Retrieved from https://www.akc.org/expert-advice/training/training-dog-therapy/

American Massage Therapy Association. (2019). Education. Retrieved from https://www.amtamassage.org/education

American Music Therapy Association. (2019). What is music therapy. Retrieved from https://www.musictherapy.org/about/musictherapy/

American Occupational Therapy Association. (2014). Occupational therapy practice framework: Domain and process (3rd ed.). *American Journal of Occupational Therapy, 68*(Supplement 1), S1–S48.

American Society for Clinical Hypnotists. (2019). Frequently asked questions about hypnosis. Retrieved from http://www.asch.net/Public/GeneralInfoonHypnosis/FAQsAboutHypnosis.aspx

American Tai Chi and Qigong Association. (2010). How to become a tai chi or qigong instructor. Retrieved from http://www.americantaichi.org/BecomeTaiChiQigongInstructor.asp

Animal Behavior Institute. (2017). Animal assisted therapy. Retrieved from https://www.animaledu.com/Programs/Animal-Assisted-Therapy

Aquatic Exercise Association. (2010). *Aquatic Fitness Professional Manual* (6th ed.). Human Kinetics.

Aquatic Therapy and Rehab Institute (n.d.) Aquatic therapeutic exercise certification. Retrieved from https://www.atri.org/atri-information/certification.html

Assefi, N., Bogart, A., Goldberg, J., & Buchwald, D. (2008). Reiki for the treatment of fibromyalgia: A randomized controlled trial. *Journal of Alternative and Complementary Medicine, 14*(9), 1115-1122. https://doi.org/10.1089/acm.2008.0068

Association of Accredited Naturopathic Medical Colleges. (2017). The six principles. Retrieved from https://aanmc.org/6-principles/

Bach, E. (2019). The 38 Bach flower remedies. Retrieved from http://www.bachflower.com/original-bach-flower-remedies/

Berman, B. M., Langevin, H. M., Witt, C. M., & Dubner, R. (2010). Acupuncture for chronic low back pain. *The New England Journal of Medicine, 363*(5), 454–461. https://doi.org/10.1056/NEJMct0806114

Bialosky, J. E., Bishop, M. D., Robinson, M. E., Zeppieri, G., & George, S. Z. (2009). Spinal manipulative therapy has an immediate effect on thermal pain sensitivity in people with low back pain: A randomized controlled trial. *Physical Therapy, 89*(12), 1292-1303. https://doi.org/10.2522/ptj.20090058

Bigley, J., Griffiths, P. D., Prydderch, A., Romanowski, C. A. J., Miles, L., Lidiard, H., & Hoggard, N. (2010). Neurolinguistic programming used to reduce the need for anaesthesia in claustrophobic patients undergoing MRI. *The British Journal of Radiology, 83*(986), 113-117. https://doi.org/10.1259/bjr/14421796

Binder, A., Parr, G., Hazleman, B., & Fitton-Jackson, S. (1984). Pulsed electromagnetic field therapy of persistent rotator cuff tendinitis. A double-blind controlled assessment. *Lancet*, (8379), 695-698. https://doi.org/10.1016/S0140-6736(84)92219-0

Biofeedback Certification International Alliance. (2019). Biofeedback and neurofeedback certification. Retrieved from https://www.bcia.org/i4a/pages/index.cfm?pageid=3636

Bridgett, R., Klose, P., Duffield, R., Mydock, S., & Lauche, R. (2018). Effects of cupping therapy in amateur and professional athletes: Systematic review of randomized controlled trials. *Journal of Alternative and Complementary Medicine, 24*(3), 208-219. https://doi.org/10.1089/acm.2017.0191

Brody, L. T., & Geigle, P. R. (2009). *Aquatic exercise for rehabilitation and training.* Human Kinetics.

Brunner, D., Abramovitch, A., & Etherton, J. (2017). A yoga program for cognitive enhancement. *PLoS One, 12*(8), e0182366. https://doi.org/10.1371/journal.pone.0182366

Canadian Paediatric Society. (1990). Megavitamin and megamineral therapy in childhood. *Canadian Medical Association Journal, 143*(1), 1009-1013.

Carroll, L. M., Volpe, D., Morris, M. E., Saunders, J., & Clifford, A. M. (2017). Aquatic exercise therapy for people with Parkinson's disease: A randomized controlled trial. *Archives of Physical Medicine and Rehabilitation, 98*(4), 631-638. https://doi.org/10.1016/j.apmr.2016.12.006

Castro-Sanchez, A. M., Lara-Palomo, I. C., Mataran-Penarrocha, G. A., Saavedra-Hernandez, M., Perez-Marmol, J. M., & Aguilar-Ferrandiz, M. E. (2016). Benefits of craniosacral therapy in patients with chronic low back pain: A randomized controlled trial. *Journal of Alternative and Complementary Medicine, 22*(8), 650-657. https://doi.org/10.1089/acm.2016.0068

Chabot, J., Beauchet, O., Fung, S., & Peretz, O. (2019). Decreased risk of falls in patients attending music sessions on an acute geriatric ward: Results from a retrospective cohort study. *BMC Complementary and Alternative Medicine, 19*(1), 1-7. https://doi.org/10.1186/s12906-019-2484-x

Chancellor, B., Duncan, A., & Chatterjee, A. (2014). Art therapy for Alzheimer's disease and other dementias. *Journal of Alzheimer's Disease, 39*(1), 1-11. https://doi.org/10.3233/JAD-131295

Chang, M. Y., Chen, C. H., Huang, K. F. (2008). Effects of music therapy on the psychological health of women during pregnancy. *Journal of Clinical Nursing, 17*(19), 2580-2587. https://doi.org/10.1111/j.1365-2702.2007.02064.x

Chellew, K., Evans, P., Fornes-Vives, J., Perez, G., & Garcia-Banda, G. (2015). The effectiveness of progressive muscle relaxation on daily cortisol secretion. *Stress, 18*(5), 538-544. https://doi.org/10.3109/10253890.2015.1053454

Chou, R., Qaseem, A., Snow, V., Casey, D., Cross, J. T. Jr., Shekelle, P., & Owens, D. K. (2007). Diagnosis and treatment of low back pain: A joint clinical practice guideline from the American College of Physicians and the American Pain Society. *Annals of Internal Medicine, 147*(7), 478–491. https://doi.org/10.7326/0003-4819-147-7-200710020-00006

Church, D. (2012). The EFT mini-manual. Retrieved from http://www.eftuniverse.com/images/pdf_files/EFTMiniManual.pdf

Cleveland Clinic. (n.d.) Aquatic rehabilitation. Retrieved from https://my.clevelandclinic.org/departments/rehabilitation/services/aquatic

Cleveland Clinic. (2014). Feel your best with functional medicine. Retrieved from https://health.clevelandclinic.org/feel-your-best-with-functional-medicine/

Cleveland Clinic. (2019). Guided imagery. Retrieved from https://my.clevelandclinic.org/departments/wellness/integrative/treatments-services/guided-imagery

Clond, M. (2016). Emotional freedom techniques for anxiety: A systematic review with meta-analysis. *The Journal of Nervous and Mental Disease, 204*(5), 388-395. https://doi.org/10.1097/NMD.0000000000000483

Cohen, M. M. (2004). CAM practitioners and regular doctors: Is integration possible? *The Medical Journal of Australia, 180*(12), 645-646. https://doi.org/10.5694/j.1326-5377.2004.tb06131.x

Corvillo, I., Varela, E., Armijo, F., Alvarez-Badillo, A., Armijo, O., & Maraver, F. (2017). Efficacy of aquatic therapy for multiple sclerosis: a systematic review. *European Journal of Physical and Rehabilitation Medicine, 53*(6), 944-952. https://doi.org/10.23736/S1973-9087.17.04570-1

Davis, T. (2017). Art therapy exhibitions: Exploitation or advocacy? *AMA Journal of Ethics, 19*(1), 98-106. https://doi.org/10.1001/journalofethics.2017.19.1.imhl1-1701

De Groot, M. (2001). Acupuncture: Complications, contraindications and informed consent. *Forsch Komplementärmed Klass Naturheilkd, 8*(5), 256-262. https://doi.org/10.1159/000057235

De Loecker W., Cheng N., & Delport P. H. (1990). Effects of pulsed electromagnetic fields on membrane transport. In: M. E. O'Connor, R. H. C. Bentall, J. C. Monahan (Eds.), *Emerging Electromagnetic Medicine* (45-57). Springer. https://doi.org/10.1007/978-1-4612-3386-2_3

Di, Y. M., May, B. H., Zhang, A. L., Zhou, I. W., Worsnop, C., & Xue, C. C. (2014). A meta-analysis of ear-acupuncture, ear-acupressure and auriculotherapy for cigarette smoking cessation. *Drug and Alcohol Dependence, 142*, 14-23. https://doi.org/10.1016/j.drugalcdep.2014.07.002

Edwards, M. K., & Loprinzi, P. D. (2018). Comparative effects of meditation and exercise on physical and psychosocial health outcomes: A review of randomized controlled trials. *Postgraduate Medicine, 130*(2), 222-228. https://doi.org/10.1080/00325481.2018.1409049

Elkina, T. N., Zakharova, L. N., Evstropov, A. N., Marinkin, I. O., Nesina, I. A., Liutkevich, A. A., Khudonogova, Z. P., Sholar, M. V., Pustovetova, M. G., Grachev, V. I., Gribanova, O. A., & Tatarenko, I. A. (2013). The experience with the application of selective polarized chromotherapy in the clinical practice. *Vopr Kurotol Fizioter Lech Fiz Kult, 6*, 42-47.

Esmel-Esmel, N., Tomas-Esmel, E., Tous-Andreu, M., Bove-Ribe, A., & Jimenez-Herrera, M. (2017). Reflexology and polysomnography: Changes in cerebral wave activity induced by reflexology promote N1 and N2 sleep stages. *Complementary Therapies in Clinical Practice, 28*, 54-64. https://doi.org/10.1016/j.ctcp.2017.05.003

Eum, Y., & Yim, J. (2015). Literature and art therapy in post-stroke psychological disorders. *The Tohoku Journal of Experimental Medicine, 235*(1), 17-23. https://doi.org/10.1620/tjem.235.17

Eye Movement Desensitization and Reprocessing International Association. (2018). What is the actual EMDR session like? Retrieved from https://www.emdria.org/page/120

Field, T. (2016). Massage therapy research review. *Complementary Therapies in Clinical Practice, 24*, 19-31. https://doi.org/10.1016/j.ctcp.2016.04.005

Foley-Nolan, D., Barry, C., Coughlan, R. J., O'Connor, P., & Roden, D. (1990). Pulsed high frequency (27MHZ) electromagnetic therapy for persistent neck pain. A double blind, placebo-controlled study of 20 patients. *Journal of Orthopaedics, 13*(4), 445-451.

Ford, A. C., Talley, N. J., Spiegel, B. M., Foxx-Orenstein, A. E., Schiller, L., Quigley, E. M., & Moayyedi, P. (2008). Effect of fibre, antispasmodics, and peppermint oil in the treatment of irritable bowel syndrome: Systematic review and meta-analysis. *British Medical Journal, 337*, a2313. https://doi.org/10.1136/bmj.a2313

Furlan, A. D., Giraldo, M., Baskwill, A., Irvin, E., & Imamura, M. (2015) Massage for low-back pain. *Cochrane Database of Systematic Reviews, 9*, CD001929. https://doi.org/10.1002/14651858.CD001929.pub3

Gade, L. (2018). Five advantages of integrative medicine. Retrieved from https://www.northwell.edu/news/five-advantages-of-integrative-medicine

Gerard, R. M. (1958). Differential effects of colored lights on psychophysiological functions. University of California, Los Angeles, Unpublished Ph.D. thesis.

Giacobbi, P., Jr., Long, D., Nolan, R., Shawley, S., Johnson, K., & Misra, R. (2018). Guided imagery targeting exercise, food cravings, and stress: A multi-modal randomized feasibility trial. *Journal of Behavioral Medicine, 41*(1), 87-98. https://doi.org/10.1007/s10865-017-9876-5

Giese, T. (2005). Complementary and alternative medicine (CAM) position paper. *The American Journal of Occupational Therapy, 59*, 653-655. https://doi.org/10.5014/ajot.59.6.653

Giggins, O. M., Persson, U. M., & Caulfield, B. (2013). Biofeedback in rehabilitation. *Journal of NeuroEngineering and Rehabilitation, 10*, 60. https://doi.org/10.1186/1743-0003-10-60

Gilmer, M. J., Baudino, M. N., Tielsch Goddard, A., Vickers, D. C., & Akard, T. F. (2016). Animal-assisted therapy in pediatric palliative care. *The Nursing Clinics of North America, 51*(3), 381-395. https://doi.org/10.1016/j.cnur.2016.05.007

Goldberg, A. (2000). Orange peel, bitter. In: M. Blumenthal, A. Goldberg, & J. Brinckmann (Eds.), *Herbal medicine: Expanded Commission E monographs* (pp. 287-289). Integrative Medicine Communications.

Gomez-Gallego, M., & Gomez-Garcia, J. (2017). Music therapy and Alzheimer's disease: Cognitive, psychological, and behavioural effects. *Neurologia, 32*(5), 300-308. https://doi.org/10.1016/j.nrl.2015.12.003

Gong, H., Ni, C., Shen, X., Wu, T., & Jiang, C. (2015). Yoga for prenatal depression: A systematic review and meta-analysis. *BMC Psychiatry, 15*, 14. https://doi.org/10.1186/s12888-015-0393-1

Gordon, G. A. (2007). Designed electromagnetic pulsed therapy: Clinical applications. *Journal of Cellular Physiology, 212*(3), 579-582. https://doi.org/10.1002/jcp.21025

Gotter, A. (2017). Cranial sacral therapy. Retrieved from https://www.healthline.com/health/cranial-sacral-therapy

Groessl, E. J., Liu, L., Chang, D. G., Wetherell, J. L., Bormann, J. E., Atkinson, J. H., Baxi, S., Schmalzl, L. (2017). Yoga for military veterans with chronic low back pain: A randomized clinical trial. *American Journal of Preventive Medicine, 53*(5), 599-608. https://doi.org/10.1016/j.amepre.2017.05.019

Hasan, F. M., Zagarins, S. E., Pischke, K. M., Saiyed, S., Bettencourt, A. M., Beal, L., Macys, D., Aurora, S., & McCleary, N. (2014). Hypnotherapy is more effective than nicotine replacement therapy for smoking cessation: Results of a randomized controlled trial. *Complementary Therapies in Medicine, 22*(1), 1-8. https://doi.org/10.1016/j.ctim.2013.12.012

Hendriks, T., De Jong, J., & Cramer, H. (2017). The effects of yoga on positive mental health among healthy adults: A systematic review and meta-analysis. *Journal of Alternative and Complementary Medicine, 23*(7), 505-517. https://doi.org/10.1089/acm.2016.0334

Hilton, L., Hempel, S., Ewing, B. A., Apaydin, E., Xenakis, L., Newberry, S., Colaiaco, B., Ruelaz Maher, A., Shanman, R. M., Sorbero, M. E., & Maglione, M. A. (2017). Mindfulness meditation for chronic pain: Systematic review and meta-analysis. *Annals of Behavioral Medicine, 51*(2), 199-213. https://doi.org/10.1007/s12160-016-9844-2

Hinman, R. S., McCrory, P., Pirotta, M., Relf, I., Forbes, A., Crossley, K. M., Williamson, E., Kyriakides, M., Novy, K., Metcalf, B. R., Harris, A., Reddy, P., Conaghan, P. G., & Bennell, K. L. (2014). Acupuncture for chronic knee pain: A randomized clinical trial. *Journal of the American Medical Association, 312*(13), 1313–1322. https://doi.org/10.1001/jama.2014.12660

Ho, S. S. M., Kwong, A. N. L., Wan, K. W. S., Ho, R. M. L., & Chow, K. M. (2017). Experiences of aromatherapy massage among adult female cancer patients: A qualitative study. *Journal of Clinical Nursing, 26*(23-24), 4519-4526. https://doi.org/10.1111/jocn.13784

Hyland, M. E., Geraghty, A. W., Joy, O. E., & Turner, S. I. (2006). Spirituality predicts outcome independently of expectancy following flower essence self-treatment. *Journal of Psychosomatic Research, 60*(1), 53-58. https://doi.org/10.1016/j.jpsychores.2005.06.073

Ikemata, S., & Momose, Y. (2017). Effects of a progressive muscle relaxation intervention on dementia symptoms, activities of daily living, and immune function in group home residents with dementia in Japan. *Japan Journal of Nursing Science, 14*(2), 135-145. https://doi.org/10.1111/jjns.12147

International Cupping Therapy Association. (n.d.). Contemporary cupping methods certification program. Retrieved from https://www.cuppingtherapy.org/pages/ccm.htm

International Iridology Practitioners Association (n.d.). How to become an IIPA certified iridologist. Retrieved from https://www.iridologyassn.org/certified-iridologist-requirements

International Neurolinguistic Programming Center. (2018). What is neurolinguistic programming and why to learn it. Retrieved from https://inlpcenter.org/what-is-neuro-linguistic-programming-nlp/

Jacobson, A. F., Umberger, W. A., Palmieri, P. A., Alexander, T. S., Myerscough, R. P., Draucker, C. B., Steudte-Schmiedgen, S., & Kirschbaum, C. (2016). Guided imagery for total knee replacement: A randomized, placebo-controlled pilot study. *Journal of Alternative and Complementary Medicine, 22*(7), 563-575. https://doi.org/10.1089/acm.2016.0038

Jakel, A., & Von Hauenschild, P. (2012). A systematic review to evaluate the clinical benefits of craniosacral therapy. *Complementary Therapies in Medicine, 20*(6), 456-465. https://doi.org/10.1016/j.ctim.2012.07.009

Janson, M. (2006). Orthomolecular medicine: The therapeutic use of dietary supplements for anti-aging. *Clinical Interventions in Aging, 1*(3), 261-265.

Jimenez-Morgan, S., & Molina-Mora, J. A. (2017). Effect of heart rate variability biofeedback on sport performance, a systematic review. *Applied Psychophysiology and Biofeedback, 42*(3), 235-245. https://doi.org/10.1007/s10484-017-9364-2

Karunaratne, M. (2010). Neuro-linguistic programming and application in treatment of phobias. *Complementary Therapies in Clinical Practice, 16*(4), 203-207. https://doi.org/10.1016/j.ctcp.2010.02.003

Kiecolt-Glaser, J. K., Graham, J. E., Malarkey, W. B., Porter, K., Lemeshow, S., & Glaser, R. (2008). Olfactory influences on mood and autonomic, endocrine, and immune function. *Psychoneuroendocrinology, 33*(3), 328–339. https://doi.org/10.1016/j.psyneuen.2007.11.015

Kiefer, D. (2016a). What is homeopathy? Retrieved from https://www.webmd.com/balance/what-is-homeopathy

Kiefer, D. (2016b). What is naturopathic medicine? Retrieved from https://www.webmd.com/balance/guide/what-is-naturopathic-medicine

Kim, T. H. M., Pascual-Leone, J., Johnson, J., & Tamim, H. (2016). The mental-attention tai chi effect with older adults. *BMC Psychology, 4*, 29. https://doi.org/10.1186/s40359-016-0137-0

Kobayashi, S., & Koitabashi, K. (2016). Effects of progressive muscle relaxation on cerebral activity: An fMRI investigation. *Complementary Therapies in Medicine, 26*, 33-39. https://doi.org/10.1016/j.ctim.2016.02.010

Kukimoto, Y., Ooe, N., & Ideguchi, N. (2017). The effects of massage therapy on pain and anxiety after surgery: A systematic review and meta-analysis. *Pain Management Nursing, 18*(6), 378-390. https://doi.org/10.1016/j.pmn.2017.09.001

Kundu, A., Lin, Y., Oron, A. P., Doorenbos, A. Z. (2015). Reiki therapy for postoperative oral pain in pediatric patients: Pilot data from a double-blind, randomized clinical trial. *Complementary Therapies in Clinical Practice, 20*(1), 21-25. https://doi.org/10.1016/j.ctcp.2013.10.010

Lan, C., Chen, S. Y., Wong, M. K., & Lai, J. S. (2013). Tai chi chuan exercise for patients with cardiovascular disease. *Evidence-Based Complementary and Alternative Medicine,*2013. https://doi.org/10.1155/2013/983208

Lauche, R., Peng, W., Ferguson, C., Cramer, H., Frawley, J., Adams, J., & Sibbritt, D. (2017). Efficacy of tai chi and qigong for the prevention of stroke and stroke risk factors. *Medicine, 96*(45), e8517. https://doi.org/10.1097/MD.0000000000008517

Lauche, R., Spitzer, J., Schwahn, B., Ostermann, T., Bernardy, K., Cramer, H., Dobos, G., & Langhorst, J. (2016). Efficacy of cupping therapy in patients with the fibromyalgia syndrome-a randomised placebo controlled trial. *Scientific Reports, 6*(2016), 37316. https://doi.org/10.1038/srep37316

Lee, S. H., Kim, J. Y., Yeo, S., Kim, S. H., & Lim, S. (2015). Meta-analysis of massage therapy on cancer pain. *Integrative Cancer Therapies, 14*(4), 297-304. https://doi.org/10.1177/1534735415572885

Li, J. Q., Guo, W., Sun, Z. G., Huang, Q. S., Lee, E. Y., Wang, Y., & Yao, X. D. (2017). Cupping therapy for treating knee osteoarthritis: The evidence from systematic review and meta-analysis. *Complementary Therapies in Clinical Practice, 28*, 152-160. https://doi.org/10.1016/j.ctcp.2017.06.003

Linde, K., Allais, G., Brinkhaus, B., Manheimer, E., Vickers, A., & White, A. R. (2009). Acupuncture for tension-type headache. *Cochrane Database of Systematic Reviews, 1*(CD007587). https://doi.org/10.1002/14651858.CD007587

Liu, X., Miller, Y. D., Burton, N. W., Chang, J. H., & Brown, W. J. (2011). Qi-gong mind-body therapy and diabetes control. A randomized controlled trial. *American Journal of Preventive Medicine, 41*(2), 152-158. https://doi.org/10.1016/j.amepre.2011.04.007

Macznik, A., Schneiders, A., Athens, J., & Sullivan, S. (2017). Does acupressure hit the mark? A three-arm randomized placebo-controlled trial of acupressure for pain and anxiety relief in athletes with acute musculoskeletal sports injuries. *Clinical Journal of Sport Medicine, 27*(4), 338-343. https://doi.org/10.1097/JSM.0000000000000378

Mafetoni, R. R., & Shimo, A. K. (2016). Effects of auriculotherapy on labour pain: A randomized clinical trial. *Revista da Escola de Enfermagem da USP, 50*(5), 726-732. https://doi.org/10.1590/s0080-623420160000600003

Magna Wave. (2019). Certification. Retrieved from https://www.magnawavepemf.com/certification-faq/

Maratos, A. S., Gold, C., Wang, X., Crawford, M. J. (2008). Music therapy for depression. *Cochrane Database Systematic Reviews, 23*(1), CD004517.

Marsden, Z., Lovell, K., Blore, D., Ali, S., & Delgadillo, J. (2018). A randomized controlled trial comparing EMDR and CBT for obsessive-compulsive disorder. *Clinical Psychology & Psychotherapy, 25*(1), e10-e18. http://doi.org/10.1002/cpp.2120

Mayo Clinic. (2017). Meditation. Retrieved from https://www.mayoclinic.org/tests-procedures/meditation/in-depth/meditation/art-20045858

Mayo Clinic. (2018). Chiropractic adjustment. Retrieved from https://www.mayoclinic.org/tests-procedures/chiropractic-adjustment/about/pac-20393513

Mayo Clinic. (2019). Biofeedback. Retrieved from https://www.mayoclinic.org/tests-procedures/biofeedback/about/pac-20384664

Mims, D., & Waddell, R. (2016). Animal assisted therapy and trauma survivors. *Journal of Evidence-Based Social Work, 13*(5), 452-457. http://doi.org/10.1080/23761407.2016.1166841

Moghimi-Hanjani, S., Mehdizadeh-Tourzani, Z., & Shoghi, M. (2015). The effect of foot reflexology on anxiety, pain, and outcomes of the labor in primigravida women. *Acta Medica Iranica, 53*(8), 507-511.

Munstedt, K., El-Safadi, S., Bruck, F., Zygmunt, M., Hackethal, A., & Tinneberg, H. R. (2005). Can iridology detect susceptibility to cancer? A prospective case-controlled study. *Journal of Alternative and Complementary Medicine, 11*(3), 515-519. http://doi.org/10.1089/acm.2005.11.515

Mutoh, T., Mutoh, T., Tsubone, H., Takada, M., Doumura, M., Ihara, M., Shimomura, H., Taki, Y., & Ihara, M. (2019). Effect of hippotherapy on gait symmetry in children with cerebral palsy: A pilot study. *Clinical and Experimental Pharmacology & Physiology, 46*(5), 506-509. http://doi.org/10.1111/1440-1681.13076

Nancarrow, S. A., Booth, A., Ariss, S., Smith, T., Enderby, P., & Roots, A. (2013). Ten principles of good interdisciplinary team work. *Human Resources for Health, 11*(19). http://doi.org/10.1186/1478-4491-11-19

National Association for Holistic Aromatherapy. (2017). Approved standards for professional aromatherapy education. Retrieved from https://naha.org/education/standards/

National Cancer Institute. (2018). Aromatherapy with essential oils (PDQ)-Patient version. Retrieved from https://www.cancer.gov/about-cancer/treatment/cam/patient/aromatherapy-pdq

National Center for Complementary and Alternative Medicine. *Expanding horizons of healthcare: Five-year strategic plan 2001-2005.* Washington DC: U.S. Department of Health and Human Services; 2000. NIH Publication No.

National Center for Complementary and Integrative Health. (2012). Chiropractic: In depth. Retrieved from https://nccih.nih.gov/health/chiropractic/introduction.htm

National Center for Complementary and Integrative Health. (2013a). Spinal manipulation for low-back pain. Retrieved from https://nccih.nih.gov/health/pain/spinemanipulation.htm

National Center for Complementary and Integrative Health. (2013b). Traditional Chinese Medicine: In depth. Retrieved from https://nccih.nih.gov/health/whatiscam/chinesemed.htm

National Center for Complementary and Integrative Health. (2016a). Acupuncture: In depth. Retrieved from https://nccih.nih.gov/health/acupuncture/introduction

National Center for Complementary and Integrative Health. (2016b). Bitter orange. Retrieved from https://nccih.nih.gov/health/bitterorange

National Center for Complementary and Integrative Health. (2016c). Massage therapy for health purposes. Retrieved from https://nccih.nih.gov/health/massage/massageintroduction.htm

National Center for Complementary and Integrative Health. (2016d). Peppermint oil. Retrieved from https://nccih.nih.gov/health/peppermintoil

National Center for Complementary and Integrative Health. (2017a). Lavender. Retrieved from https://nccih.nih.gov/health/lavender

National Center for Complementary and Integrative Health. (2017b). Naturopathy. Retrieved from https://nccih.nih.gov/health/naturopathy

National Center for Complementary and Integrative Health. (2018a). Complementary, alternative, or integrative health: What's in a name? Retrieved from https://www.nccih.nih.gov/health/complementary-alternative-or-integrative-health-whats-in-a-name

National Center for Complementary and Integrative Health. (2018b). Homeopathy. Retrieved from https://nccih.nih.gov/health/homeopathy

National Center for Complementary and Integrative Health. (2018c). Reiki. Retrieved from https://nccih.nih.gov/health/reiki-info

National Center for Complementary and Integrative Health. (2018d). Yoga: In depth. Retrieved from https://nccih.nih.gov/health/yoga/introduction.htm

National Center for Complementary and Integrative Health. (2019). Ayurvedic medicine: In depth. Retrieved from https://nccih.nih.gov/health/ayurveda/introduction.htm

National Certification Commission for Acupuncture and Oriental Medicine. (n.d.). Becoming a board-certified AOM practitioner. Retrieved from https://www.nccaom.org/certification/becoming-certified/

National Certification Commission for Acupuncture and Oriental Medicine. (2018). The NCCAOM certification in Asian bodywork therapy. Retrieved from https://www.nccaom.org/wp-content/uploads/pdf/NCCAOM%20ABT%20Certification%20Fact%20Sheet060318.pdf

National Certification Commission for Acupuncture and Oriental Medicine. (2019). NCCAOM certification handbook. Retrieved from https://www.nccaom.org/wp-content/uploads/pdf/NCCAOM%20Certification%20Handbook_Interim_12920.pdf

National Qigong Association. (n.d.). What is qigong? Retrieved from https://www.nqa.org/what-is-qigong-

Nelms, J. A., & Castel, L. (2016). A systematic review and meta-analysis of randomized and nonrandomized trials of clinical emotional freedom techniques (EFT) for the treatment of depression. *Explore, 12*(6), 416-426. https://doi.org/10.1016/j.explore.2016.08.001

Nelson, N. L., & Churilla, J. R. (2017). Massage therapy for pain and function in patients with arthritis: A systematic review of randomized controlled trials. *American Journal of Physical Medicine & Rehabilitation, 96*(9), 665-672. https://doi.org/10.1097/PHM.0000000000000712

O'Mathuna, D. P. (2016). Therapeutic touch for healing acute wounds. *Cochrane Database Systematic Review, 9,* CD002766. https://doi.org/10.1002/14651858.CD002766.pub6

Ozdelikara, A., & Tan, M. (2017). The effect of reflexology on the quality of life with breast cancer patients. *Complementary Therapies in Clinical Practice, 29,* 122-129. https://doi.org/10.1016/j.ctcp.2017.09.004

Pant, C. R., Pokharel, G. P., Curtale, F., Pokhrel, R. P., Grosse, R. N., Lepkowski, J., Muhilal, Gorstein J., Pak-Gorstein S., Atmarita, & Tilden, R. L. (1996). Impact of nutrition education and mega-dose vitamin A supplementation on the health of children in Nepal. *Bulletin of the World Health Organization, 74*(5), 533-545.

Paragas, E. D., Ng, A. T. Y., Reyes, D. V. L., & Reyes, G. A. B. (2019). Effects of chromotherapy on the cognitive ability of older adults: A quasi-experimental study. *Explore, S1550-8307*(18), 30172. https://doi.org/10.1016/j.explore.2019.01.002

Patwardhan, B., Warude, D., Pushpangadan, P., & Bhatt, N. (2005). Ayurveda and Traditional Chinese Medicine: A comparative overview. *Evidence-Based Complementary and Alternative Medicine, 2*(4), 465-473. https://doi.org/10.1093/ecam/neh140

Pelletier, K. R., & Astin, J. A. (2002). Integration and reimbursement of complementary and alternative medicine by managed care and insurance providers: 2000 update and cohort analysis. *Alternative Therapies in Health and Medicine, 8*(1), 38-44.

Pelletier, K. R., Astin, J. A., & Haskell, W. L. (1999). Current trends in the integration and reimbursement of complementary and alternative medicine by managed care organizations (MCOs) and insurance providers: 1998 update and cohort analysis. *American Journal of Health Promotion, 14*(2), 125-133. https://doi.org/10.4278/0890-1171-14.2.125

Perry, R., Terry, R., Watson, L. K., & Ernst, E. (2012). Is lavender an anxiolytic drug? A systematic review of randomised clinical trials. *Phytomedicine, 19*(8-9), 825-835. https://doi.org/10.1016/j.phymed.2012.02.013

Petersen, D. (2017). *Historical modalities I: Iridology* (17th ed.). American College of Healthcare Sciences Publishing.

Pilz, R., Hartleb, R., Konrad, G., Reininghaus, E., & Unterrainer, H. F. (2017). The role of eye movement desensitization and reprocessing (EMDR) in substance use disorders: A systematic review. *Fortschritte der Neurologie Psychiatrie, 85*(10), 584-591. https://doi.org/10.1055/s-0043-118338

Polat, H., & Erguney, S. (2017). The effect of reflexology applied to patients with chronic obstructive pulmonary disease on dyspnea and fatigue. *Rehabilitation Nursing, 42*(1), 14-21. https://doi.org/10.1002/rnj.266

Posadzki, P., Lewandowski, W., Terry, R., Ernst, E., & Stearns, A. (2012). Guided imagery for non-musculoskeletal pain: A systematic review of randomized clinical trials. *Journal of Pain and Symptom Management, 44*(1), 95-104. https://doi.org/10.1016/j.jpainsymman.2011.07.014

Przybyla, D. (2018). Chromotherapy guide: What is color therapy and how it heals your body. Retrieved from https://www.colorpsychology.org/chromotherapy/

Qigong Institute. (2019). Getting started with qigong. Retrieved from https://www.qigonginstitute.org/category/4/getting-started

Reb, A. M., Saum, N. S., Murphy, D. A., Breckenridge-Sproat, S. T., Su, X., & Bormann, J. E. (2017). Qigong in injured military service members. *Journal of Holistic Nursing, 35*(1), 10-24. https://doi.org/10.1177/0898010116638159

Riordan Clinic. (2017). Micronutrients. Retrieved from http://orthomolecular.org/nutrients/micronutrients.shtml

Rivas Neira, S., Pasqual-Marques A., Pegito Perez, I., Fernandez Cervantes, R., & Vivas Costa, J. (2017). Effectiveness of aquatic therapy vs land-based therapy for balance and pain in women with fibromyalgia: A study protocol for a randomised controlled trial. *BMC Musculoskeletal Disorders, 18*(1), 22. https://doi.org/10.1186/s12891-016-1364-5

Rivas-Suarez, S. R., Aguila-Vazquez, J., Suarez-Rodriguez, B., Vazquez-Leon, L., Casanova-Giral, M., Morales-Morales, R., & Rodriguez-Martin, B. C. (2017). Exploring the effectiveness of external use of Bach flower remedies on carpal tunnel syndrome: A pilot study. *Journal of Evidence-Based Complementary and Alternative Medicine, 22*(1), 18-24. https://doi.org/10.1177/2156587215610705

Rodriguez-Mansilla, J., Gonzalez-Lopez-Arza, M. V., Varela-Donoso, E., Montanero-Fernandez, J., Jimenez-Palomares, M., & Garrido-Ardila, E. M. (2013). Ear therapy and massage therapy in elderly people with dementia: A pilot study. *Journal of Traditional Chinese Medicine, 33*(4), 461-467. https://doi.org/10.1016/S0254-6272(13)60149-1

Rong, P., Lui, A., Zhang, J., Wang, Y., Yang, A., Li, L., Ben, H., Li, L., Liu, R., He, W., Liu, H., Huang, F., Li, X., Wu, P., & Zhu, B. (2014). An alternative therapy for drug-resistant epilepsy: Transcutaneous auricular vagus nerve stimulation. *Journal of Chinese Medicine, 127*(2), 300-304.

Ross, C. L. (2009). Integral healthcare: The benefits and challenges of integrating complementary and alternative medicine with a conventional healthcare practice. *Integrative Medicine Insights, 4*, 13-20. https://doi.org/10.4137/IMI.S2239

Scott, E. (2018). Use guided imagery for relaxation. Retrieved from https://www.verywellmind.com/use-guided-imagery-for-relaxation-3144606

Sebastian, B., & Nelms, J. (2017). The effectiveness of emotional freedom techniques in the treatment of posttraumatic stress disorder: A meta-analysis. *Explore, 13*(1), 16-25. https://doi.org/10.1016/j.explore.2016.10.001

Seyedi Chegeni, P., Gholami, M., Azargoon, A., Hossein Pour, A. H., Birjandi, M., & Norollahi, H. (2018). The effect of progressive muscle relaxation on the management of fatigue and quality of sleep in patients with chronic obstructive pulmonary disease: A randomized controlled clinical trial. *Complementary Therapies in Clinical Practice, 31*, 64-70. https://doi.org/10.1016/j.ctcp.2018.01.010

Shang, A., Huwiler-Muntener, K., Nartey, L., Juni, P., Dorig, S., Sterne, J. A., Pewsner, D., & Egger, M. (2005). Are the clinical effects of homeopathy placebo effects? Comparative study of placebo-controlled trials of homeopathy and allopathy. *The Lancet, 366*(9487), 726-732. https://doi.org/10.1016/S0140-6736(05)67177-2

Shapiro, F. (2014). The role of eye movement desensitization and reprocessing (EMDR) therapy in medicine: Addressing the psychological and physical symptoms stemming from adverse life experiences. *The Permanente Journal, 18*(1), 71-77. https://doi.org/10.7812/TPP/13-098

Siegler, M., Frange, C., Andersen, M.L., Tufik, S., & Hachul, H. (2017). Effects of Bach flower remedies on menopausal symptoms and sleep pattern: A case report. *Alternative Therapies in Health and Medicine, 23*(2), 44-48.

Sielski, R., Rief, W., & Glombiewski, J. A. (2017). Efficacy of biofeedback in chronic back pain: A meta-analysis. *International Journal of Behavioral Medicine, 24*(1), 25-41. https://doi.org/10.1007/s12529-016-9572-9

Sjoling, M., Rolleri, M., & Englund, E. (2008). Auricular acupuncture versus sham acupuncture in the treatment of women who have insomnia. *Journal of Alternative and Complementary Medicine, 14*(1), 39-46. https://doi.org/10.1089/acm.2007.0544

Smith, C. A., Armour, M., & Dahlen, H. G. (2017). Acupuncture or acupressure for induction of labour. *Cochrane Database of Systematic Reviews, 10*, CD002962. https://doi.org/10.1002/14651858.CD002962.pub4

Song, R., Grabowska, W., Park, M., Osypiuk, K., Vergara-Diaz, G. P., Bonato, P., Hausdorff, J. M., Fox, M., Sudarsky, L. R., Macklin, E., & Wayne, P. M. (2017). The impact of tai chi and qigong mind-body exercises on motor and non-motor function and quality of life in Parkinson's disease: A systematic review and meta-analysis. *Parkinsonism Related Disorders, 41*, 3-13. https://doi.org/10.1016/j.parkreldis.2017.05.019

Sorenson, L. B., Greve, T., Kreutzer, M., Pedersen, U., Nielsen, C. M., Toubro, S., & Astrup, A. (2011). Weight maintenance through behaviour modification with a cooking course or neurolinguistic programming. *Canadian Journal of Dietetic Practice and Research, 72*(4), 181-185. https://doi.org/10.3148/72.4.2011.181

Sova, R. (2012). *Introduction of aquatic therapy and rehab*, (3rd ed.). DSL, Ltd.

Stapleton, P., Bannatyne, A., Chatwin, H., Urzi, K. C., Porter, B., & Sheldon, T. (2017). Secondary psychological outcomes in a controlled trial of emotional freedom techniques and cognitive behaviour therapy in the treatment of food cravings. *Complementary Therapy Clinical Practices, 28*, 136-145. https://doi.org/10.1016/j.ctcp.2017.06.004

Stearn, N., & Swanepoel, D. W. (2006). Identifying hearing loss by means of iridology. *African Journal of Traditional, Complementary, and Alternative Medicine, 4*(2), 205-210. http://doi.org/10.4314/ajtcam.v4i2.31209

Szigethy, E. (2015). Hypnotherapy for inflammatory bowel disease across the lifespan. *American Journal of Clinical Hypnosis, 58*(1), 81-99. https://doi.org/10.1080/00029157.2015.1040112

Tabatabaee, A., Zagheri-Tafreshi, M., Rassouli, M., Amir-Aledavood, S., AlaviMajd, H., & Kazem-Farahmand, S. (2016). Effect of therapeutic touch in patients with cancer: A literature review. *Medical Archives, 70*(2), 142-147. https://doi.org/10.5455/medarh.2016.70.142-147

Tan, J., Molassiotis, A., Wang, T., & Suen, L. K. P. (2014). Adverse events of auricular therapy: A systematic review. *Evidence-Based Complementary and Alternative Medicine, 506758*, https://doi.org/10.1155/2014/506758

Tellez, A., Rodriguez-Padilla, C., Martinez-Rodriguez, J. L., Juarez-Garcia, D. M., Sanchez-Armass, O., Sanchez, T., Segura G., & Jaime-Bernal, L. (2017). Psychological effects of group hypnotherapy on breast cancer patients during chemotherapy. *American Journal of Clinical Hypnosis, 60*(1), 68-84. https://doi.org/10.1080/00029157.2016.1210497

The Auriculotherapy Certification Institute. (2014). Course study information. Retrieved from https://www.auriculotherapy.org/course-study/

The Bravewell Collaborative. (2010). Integrative medicine: Improving health care for patients and health care delivery for providers and payors. Retrieved from http://www.bravewell. org/content/pdf/IntegrativeMedicine2.pdf

The Institute for Functional Medicine. (2019). The functional medicine approach. Retrieved from https://www.ifm.org/functional-medicine/what-is-functional-medicine/

The International Center for Reiki Training. (2019). What is reiki? Retrieved from https:// www.reiki.org/faq/whatisreiki.html

Thrane, S., & Cohen, S. M. (2015). Effect of reiki therapy on pain and anxiety in adults: An in-depth literature review of randomized trials with effect size calculations. *Pain Management Nursing, 15*(4), 897-908. https://doi.org/10.1016/j.pmn.2013.07.008

Tillotson, A. K. (2001). *The one Earth herbal sourcebook: Everything you need to know about Chinese, Western, and Ayurvedic herbal treatments.* Kensington Publishing Corporation.

Travers, B. G., Mason, A. H., Mrotek, L. A., Ellertson, A., Dean, D. C., Engel, C., Gomez, A., Dadalko, O. I., & McLaughlin, K. (2018). Biofeedback-based, videogame balance training in autism. *Journal of Autism and Developmental Disorders, 48*(1), 163-175. https://doi. org/10.1007/s10803-017-3310-2

Ulug, N., Yilmaz, O. T., Kara, M., & Ozcakar, L. (2018). Effects of pilates and yoga in patients with chronic neck pain: A sonographic study. *Journal of Rehabilitation Medicine, 50*(1), 80-85. https://doi.org/10.2340/16501977-2288

University of California at Los Angeles Integrative Medicine. (2019). Acupressure for beginners. Retrieved from https://exploreim.ucla.edu/self-care/acupressure-and-common-acupressure-points/

University of Michigan Medicine. (2018). Stress management: Doing progressive muscle relaxation. Retrieved from https://www.uofmhealth.org/health-library/uz2225

University of Minnesota. (2016). How does reflexology work? Retrieved from https://www.takingcharge.csh.umn.edu/explore-healing-practices/reflexology/ how-does-reflexology-work

Upledger Institute International. (2019). Certification programs. Retrieved from https://www. upledger.com/therapies/certification-programs.php

Vadala, M., Vallelunga, A., Palmieri, L., Palmieri, B., Morales-Medina, J. C., & Iannitti, T. (2015). Mechanisms and therapeutic applications of electromagnetic therapy in Parkinson's disease. *Behavior and Brain Function, 11*, 26. https://doi.org/10.1186/s12993-015-0070-z

Valiente-Gomez, A., Moreno-Alcazar, A., Treen, D., Cedron, C., Colom, F., Perez, V., & Amann, B. L. (2017). EMDR beyond PTSD: A systematic literature review. *Frontiers in Psychology, 8*, 1668. https://doi.org/10.3389/fpsyg.2017.01668

Vickers, A., Zollman, C., & Lee, R. (2001). Herbal medicine. *Western Journal of Medicine, 175*(2), 125-128.

Victoria State Government. (2018). Ayurveda. Retrieved from https://www.betterhealth.vic.gov. au/health/ConditionsAndTreatments/ayurveda

Wachholtz, A. B., Malone, C. D., & Pargament, K. I. (2017). Effect of different meditation types on migraine headache medication use. *Behavioral Medicine, 43*(1), 1-8. https://doi.org/10.1 080/08964289.2015.1024601

Wang, C., Schmid, C. H., Fielding, R. A., Harvey, W. F., Reid, K. F., Price, L. L., Driban, J. B., Kalish, R., Rones, R., & McAlindon, T. (2018). Effect of tai chi versus aerobic exercise for fibromyalgia: comparative effective randomized controlled trial. *The British Medical Journal, 360*, k851. https://doi.org/10.1136/bmj.k851

Wang, Y. T., Qi, Y., Tang, F. Y., Li, F. M., Li, Q. H., Xu, C. P., Xie, G. P., & Sun, H. T. (2017). The effect of cupping therapy for low back pain: A meta-analysis based on existing randomized controlled trials. *Journal of Back and Musculoskeletal Rehabilitation, 30*(6), 1187-1195. https://doi.org/10.3233/BMR-169736

Weintraub, M. (2004). Magnetotherapy: Historical background with a stimulating future. *Critical Reviews™ in Physical and Rehabilitation Medicine, 16*(2), 95-108. https://doi.org/10.1615/CritRevPhysRehabilMed.v16.i2.20

Wetzler, G., Roland, M., Fryer-Dietz, S., & Dettmann-Ahern, D. (2017). Craniosacral therapy and visceral manipulation: A new treatment intervention for concussion recovery. *Medical Acupuncture, 29*(4), 239-248. https://doi.org/10.1089/acu.2017.1222

Witt, C. M., Jena, S., Brinkhaus, B., Liecker, B., Wegscheider, K., & Willich, S. N. (2006). Acupuncture for patients with chronic neck pain. *Pain, 125*(1–2), 98–106. https://doi.org/10.1016/j.pain.2006.05.013

Wong, C. (2017). The benefits and uses of acupressure. Retrieved from https://www.verywellhealth.com/the-benefits-of-acupressure-88702

Wong, C. (2019). Cupping therapy overview, benefits, and side effects. Retrieved from https://www.verywellhealth.com/cupping-for-pain-88933

Wood, E., Ricketts, T., & Parry, G. (2018). EMDR as a treatment for long-term depression: A feasibility study. *Psychology and Psychotherapy, 91*(1), 63-78. https://doi.org/10.1111/papt.12145

Wood, W., Fields, B., Rose, M., & McLure, M. (2017). Animal-assisted therapies and dementia: A systematic mapping review using the Lived Environment Life Quality (LELQ) model. *American Journal of Occupational Therapy, 71*(5). https://doi.org/10.5014/ajot.2017.027219

Xiang, Y., Lu, L., Chen, X., & Wen, Z. (2017). Does tai chi relieve fatigue? A systematic review and meta-analysis of randomized controlled trials. *PLOS ONE, 12*(4), e0174872. https://doi.org/10.1371/journal.pone.0174872

Yoga Alliance. (2018). Spirit of the standards. Retrieved from https://www.yogaalliance.org/Credentialing/Standards/200-HourStandards

Yousuf Azeemi, S. T., & Mohsin-Raza, S. (2005). A critical analysis of chromotherapy and its scientific evolution. *Evidence-Based Complementary and Alternative Medicine, 2*(4), 481-488. https://doi.org/10.1093/ecam/neh137

Zarabi-Smith, N. (2013). *L.E.D. Light therapy: Explore beyond limitations.* The Quantum Academies.

Zech, N., Hansen, E., Bernardy, K., & Hauser, W. (2017). Efficacy, acceptability and safety of guided imagery/hypnosis in fibromyalgia - A systematic review and meta-analysis of randomized controlled trials. *European Journal of Pain, 21*(2), 217-227. https://doi.org/10.1002/ejp.933

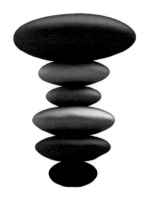

Index

Printed in the United States
by Baker & Taylor Publisher Services